# DEVELOPING CHILDREN'S SPEECH, LANGUAGE AND COMMUNICATION THROUGH STORIES AND DRAMA

Using drama activities based on a range of classic and modern stories, this inspiring resource equips SENCOs, primary-school teachers and speech and language therapists alike with simple, practical and effective tools to improve children's speech, language and communication. Key features include the following: a huge range of activities so that the resource can be used in focused support for those with SGBPN or in mixed-ability classrooms; topical links to the English programmes of study so that activities support core curriculum learning; and distinct sections for Key Stage 1 and Key Stage 2 make the book relevant from Reception to Year 6. Unlike alternative resources, this book uses drama techniques to address speech, language and communication needs, and it can be used for both therapy and mainstream primary education.

**Jodi Lea-Trowman** practised as a Highly Specialist Speech and Language Therapist within the NHS for many years before founding www.lovetocommunicate.co.uk. Jodi has significant experience training staff in primary and secondary schools and working directly with children and young people.

# DEVELOPING CHILDREN'S SPEECH, LANGUAGE AND COMMUNICATION THROUGH STORIES AND DRAMA

Jodi Lea-Trowman
(MRCSLT, MASLTIP, MHPC)

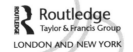

Routledge
Taylor & Francis Group

LONDON AND NEW YORK

First published 2018
by Routledge
2 Park Square, Milton Park, Abingdon, Oxon OX14 4RN

and by Routledge
711 Third Avenue, New York, NY 10017

*Routledge is an imprint of the Taylor & Francis Group, an informa business*

© 2018 Jodi Lea-Trowman

*British Library Cataloguing-in-Publication Data*
A catalogue record for this book is available from the British Library

*Library of Congress Cataloging-in-Publication Data*
A catalog record for this book has been requested

ISBN: 978-1-911186-13-7 (pbk)
ISBN: 978-1-315-17281-1 (ebk)

Typeset in DIN Pro
by Apex CoVantage, LLC

# CONTENTS

# Contents

# ACKNOWLEDGEMENTS

This book has been a long time in the making and was always just an idea stored away in the depths of my mind in the category 'maybe one day.' I would like to express my gratitude to my amazing parents and sister for their continuous support in all I do. They have instilled in me that I can do anything I put my mind to and to always 'go for it,' which I eventually did . . .

I give sincere thanks to the talented drama practitioners that I worked alongside from 2007 to 2009. We went on an amazing journey together, and they inspired me, taught me new ways of communicating and practicing, and most importantly . . . helped me become a better therapist.

Thanks goes to Adam Annand from London Bubble Theatre, who has continued to see the benefit of this kind of work and has continued to share his expertise with me since the project ended.

I would like to acknowledge, with gratitude, the love and support I have received from my very own happy ever after – my fabulous husband, Ward Trowman . . . thank you . . . I couldn't have done it without you.

Finally, as a storyteller, I know all about that magic rule of three. The Three Pigs, Three Bears, three wishes . . . My three very special little people: Rafferty, Starla and Sunny – thank you for being my magic three, my inspiration and my world . . .

# ABOUT THE AUTHOR

Jodi Lea-Trowman is a Highly Specialist Speech and Language Therapist practicing since 2002. She worked within the NHS for 12 years and, following this, established her own independent practice – 'Love to Communicate' – based in London and Brighton in 2013.

The author's experience with speech and language and drama began in 2007. She was designated as the lead therapist for an innovative project in Lewisham, funded mainly by Arts Council England (ACE) London.

The project focus was particularly on partnership working between health and the arts and developing children's communication skills through drama.

The project combined the speech and language therapist's (SALT) knowledge of speech and language with the creativity and imagination of the drama practitioners to create an environment where the children's speaking, listening and confidence would develop.

Both assessment results and anecdotal evidence showed increased language skills, communication skills and confidence in children (for further information on this project, the complete evaluation can be accessed: O'Neill, 2007–2009, Evaluation of Speak Out).

The project influenced Jodi's practice as a Speech and Language Therapist, and she continued to apply her learning and experience from this project into her own therapy.

She has developed sessions integrating drama techniques and speech and language to focus on developing children's speech, language and communication skills.

Her practice has evolved and is now far more focused on experiencing language and learning and making language come alive through storytelling and drama.

# INTRODUCTION

The following programme is based on the amalgamation of two practices that naturally complement and influence each other: Communication and Drama.

Drama enables us to explore stories/situations and language in a creative environment and puts learning and language into a purposeful and meaningful context – vitally important for children.

We are surrounded by stories throughout our lives. They inspire us, entertain us and enhance our understanding of the world.

Our need for stories shows how we need to understand patterns of life, and, as Bruner (1996) has stated, we live our lives and shape our identities through stories.

Stories are the way to reach out to children and emotionally connect, and experiencing and exploring stories with scaffolding will enable children to embed the learning of language and communication skills more effectively.

The session plans within this programme provide fun and accessible sessions, focusing on building language and communication skills around topics and stories that children are covering within their curriculum.

It can be used as a pre-teaching or post-teaching (review/embedding) tool and can be used for children with speech, language and communication need (SLCN); for children who need additional review/recap and exposure to language and learning; or simply as a teaching tool to complement the story, topic and themes being learned in the classroom.

This book firstly provides some theory around drama and communication and the fundamentals behind running the sessions and activities within them.

The 'practice' part is then presented through two sections:

Chapters two and three provide ready-made sessions for Early Years and Key Stage 1, and Chapter four provides activities to build into sessions for Key Stage 2.

# Chapter one
# THE THEORY

## How the programme works

### Objective

This programme is not to develop children into actors and actresses. It is designed to help them develop their language and communication skills and to access parts of the curriculum. They experience stories and topics through innovative games and activities and through guided discussion.

Sessions should enable them to make sense of the world and to go on a creative journey that facilitates them accessing and retaining learning of many skills.

### Flexibility

This programme has been designed to be as flexible as possible – both for the use of the practitioners and for the children experiencing the programme.

Activities can be changed to suit the stories or topics the practitioner is covering, and sessions can be changed and added to. . . .

For example . . . 'The Shopping Basket' (by John Burningham) session has a focus activity around bullying . . . this activity could easily be placed in a session based on the story 'Frog and the Stranger' (by Max Velthuijs).

Choosing sessions can be influenced through various factors. It may be that a story being read/covered in class is used in the sessions as a pre-/post-teaching strategy, or a story familiar to the children could be used at that time to then work on language and communication skills.

It could be that a particular topic is being covered in class – e.g. healthy vs. non-healthy foods – and the practitioner decides to use 'The Very Hungry Caterpillar' story to reflect this topic.

The Key Stage 2 section of this programme is far more topic-based and gives examples of activities that can be used for a variety of stories and topics.

The programme isn't linear, and sessions can be chosen according to what story the practitioner wants to facilitate.

Equally, some activities may suit other stories/projects that the children are learning and can be adapted by the practitioners.

Each session has a framework to follow which will be the same for most sessions with the content inside the session changing.

## Who can use this programme?

Both speech and language therapists and teachers can use this programme.

In an ideal practice it should be used where both the teacher and the SALT are liaising/collaborating and even joint delivering.

If teachers are going to run sessions from this book, it is recommended that they have some experience of SLCN and liaise with a qualified speech and language therapist.

In equal terms, if a speech and language therapist is going to run sessions from this programme, best practice would be to liaise with teachers around stories/topics/ themes the children are covering in class so that the sessions they choose from this programme reflect language and learning from the children's classroom.

The programme is built around the fundamentals of delivering sessions to children with speech, language and communication need, but also the techniques can be used for all children and link into the expectations of high-quality teaching.

The national curriculum is reflected throughout the sessions, and stories that are used are linked to the curriculum and national curriculum objectives.

Sessions are designed so that the practitioner can have a session ready-made for them and to have the learning and objectives of the activities clearly outlined.

Sessions can however be added to, shortened, or changed at the discretion of the practitioner. General drama games and techniques are provided so that the practitioners also have autonomy over the sessions and can add and take away as they feel necessary to suit the children they are working with.

Sessions can also lead to children producing their own stories as their skills improve, and sessions can then evolve into reflecting the children's own learning, and they can take ownership of this.

The programme has much scope, and although sessions are outlined they are easy to adapt and change and evolve with the practitioner running them and the children participating.

The programme can be run with a whole class, with a half class, or within a small group.

The smaller the group, the more SLCN-focused the tasks can be; however, whole-class use can be beneficial in terms of the children experiencing stories and language.

## Links to national curriculum

This programme includes various aspects of the national curriculum so that participants are following objectives from the curriculum in addition to improving their speech, language and communication.

The following areas have been considered and are reflected throughout the programme:

1   *Some of the main goals set out in the new English national curriculum are reflected within the programme, including:*

- A strong focus on vocabulary

- Familiarity with key stories, traditional tales, etc.

- Having 'conversations about books'

- Oral rehearsal of ideas and sentences prior to writing.

2   *The programme aims to target the statutory requirements set out in the Spoken Language section of 'The National Curriculum in England Framework Document 2014' (covering Years 1 to 6).*[1]

## Statutory requirements

Pupils should be taught to:

- listen and respond appropriately to adults and their peers

- ask relevant questions to extend their understanding and knowledge

- use relevant strategies to build their vocabulary

- articulate and justify answers, arguments and opinions

- give well-structured descriptions, explanations and narratives for different purposes, including for expressing feelings

- maintain attention and participate actively in collaborative conversations, staying on topic and initiating and responding to comments

- use spoken language to develop understanding through speculating, hypothesising, imagining and exploring ideas

- speak audibly and fluently with an increasing command of Standard English

- participate in discussions, presentations, performances, role-play, improvisations and debates

- gain, maintain and monitor the interest of the listener(s)

- consider and evaluate different viewpoints, attending to and building on the contributions of others

- select and use appropriate registers for effective communication.

3   *The programme is reflective of the Prime Areas in Learning and Development in the 'Early Years and Foundation Stage Framework.'[2] The Communication and Language Units are reflected in particular.*

4   *The seven areas within the SEAL (Social and Emotional Aspects of Learning) curriculum are covered within different stories throughout the programme.*

- New beginnings

- Getting on and falling out

- Say 'no' to bullying

- Going for goals

- Good to be me

- Relationships

- Changes.

5  *PHSE Association divided SEAL into three core themes which are also considered in the planning of sessions:*

- Health and well-being

- Relationships

- Living in the wider world.

  PHSE education[3] equips pupils with the knowledge, understanding, skills and strategies required to live healthy, safe, productive, capable, responsible and balanced lives. (PHSE Association, 2016)

6  *Topics: all year groups from Reception to Year 6 have different topics. Schools choose which topics they are going to explore.*

  Each story and theme chosen in this particular programme will be linked with a topic so that it can be integrated into the children's curriculum.

7  *Narrative aspects within literacy curriculum: all stories chosen in this programme will be linked to one of the following categories:*

- Predictable patterned language

- Stories with familiar settings

- Stories from a range of cultures

- Traditional and fairy stories

- Stories about fantasy worlds

- Poetry

- Stories by the same author.

8  *Preparation for writing: children need to know a story before writing it . . .*

The narrative content and scaffolding within sessions provides a foundation for children before writing stories.

Pie Corbett and Julia Strong (2011) describe the 'story making process' as Imitation – Innovation – Invention.

Some sessions focus on imitation of stories, and some then work on innovation and changing parts of a known story. Finally, some sessions work on invention of own stories/answers/descriptions.

Teachers could use these sessions as building blocks before writing tasks.

9   *Pre-teaching/post-teaching:*

Sessions can be used to pre-teach vocabulary, story content, concepts and so on that are going to be introduced in the classroom.

Children with SLCN can benefit hugely from pre-teaching as they get the opportunity to hear and put into context language and learning from the session, before they are exposed to it in the classroom.

This gives them increased exposure, and they will therefore recognise words/characters/themes more effectively in the classroom.

Equally, post-teaching of the stories/topics being learned in the classroom are effective as they give children the opportunity for recap and review of language and learning, which again is extremely valuable to children with SLCN.

## Evidence

The effectiveness of drama and speech and language intervention has been investigated through various means, but it remains an area with very little in-depth research.

The author has been involved in the following research / practical experience. These projects show positive outcomes for children who participated in the interventions.

## 'Speak Out' project

The 'Speak Out' project previously mentioned was evaluated[4] and demonstrated a significant increase in children's scores (there was not a control group in this evaluation to compare progress made).

Eighteen schools signed up for the project. Twenty children were chosen by school staff (those identified with some degree of speech, language and communication need) and split into two groups of ten.

These groups then had a year of weekly groups lasting 45 minutes. The sessions were led by the drama practitioner and the speech and language therapist.

A pre- and post-screen of children's language skills was carried out with the Assessment of Comprehension and Expression 6–11 years (Adams, Coke, Crutchley, Hesketh, and Reeves, 2001). The areas chosen for assessment and analysis were sentence comprehension, naming and narrative.

*Post-screener results showed:*

Sentence Comprehension:

67.5% of children assessed: increased scaled scores in this area

Naming:

40.5% of children assessed: increased scaled scores in this area

Narrative Propositions:

70.2% of children assessed: increased scaled scores in this area

Narrative syntax/discourse:

48.6% of children assessed: increased scaled scores in this area

(O'Neill, 2007–2009)

Jodi Lea-Trowman analysed the data and obtained information on which children responded the most significantly to the intervention in terms of their specific SLCN.

The children who responded the most significantly and increased scaled scores by at least 1 were those with English as an additional language, children with language delay and those children with poor confidence and mild SLCN.

Those with more complex SLCN such as language disorders and social communication difficulties, although they responded to the intervention, did not show as much significant change – most likely due to the complex nature of their need.

Some children with social communication difficulties, however (although their language scores may not have significantly changed), displayed improvement in social skills and confidence within a group. Anecdotal evidence was collected for these children from teachers and parents, and, often, improved outcomes were observed.

## Independent speech and drama project

Following 'Speak Out,' speech and language therapist Jodi-Lea Trowman carried out sessions with a Year 1 group consisting of six children, in a primary school.

These groups ran for six weeks, for 45 minutes each session.

The speech and language therapist and a teaching assistant facilitated the sessions. No drama practitioner was present, and the groups were based on knowledge and experience that the speech and language therapist had gained through her previous work.

Pre- and post-assessment of children's narrative skills were carried out using the 'Peter and the Cat' assessment Leitáo and Allan (2004). This is a task that obtains a descriptive profile of the child's development of key narrative competencies.

Children listened to the 'Peter and the Cat' story accompanied by pictures and were then asked to retell the stories with the pictures as a support. Their story was then analysed by looking at its:

Structure, content, vocabulary, connectors, referencing (use of pronouns: she/Peter), adverbials, and story register (use of tense / narrative features).

The participant's scores improved across all areas (however, improvement in using connectors was minimal). The children all enjoyed the sessions, and their confidence and participation visibly improved as the sessions progressed.

## 'Speech Bubbles'

Following 'Speak Out,' the London Bubble Theatre Company could see the advantages of the project for children with speech, language and communication needs, and it set up a new programme based on some of the learning the drama practitioners had acquired. This was named the 'Speech Bubbles' programme. It is a drama-oriented school-based intervention for children with identified speech, language and communication needs in Key Stage 1.

It is distinctive in working with the whole body, putting children's own narrated stories at the centre of the workshops and building young children's confidence without immediate pressure to speak.

It runs weekly for 20 weeks within schools in disadvantaged areas, using trained drama practitioners paired with the schools' own familiar learning support staff (Price, 2016). Speech and language therapists are not involved in the planning or running of these groups or programme.

A preliminary evaluation of the effectiveness of the 'Speech Bubbles' programme was conducted in 2015 and 2016 by Dr Heather Price (Psychological Research Group, UEL) and statistical analysis undertaken by Eric Ansong (School of Social Sciences, UEL).[5]

The Communication Trust's Primary Speech, Language and Communication progression tool[6] was used to review the progress of the participants in selected Southwark schools in 2015–2016. It was shown that the participants made good progress in their speech, language and communication development.

In most cases, the progress made lifted the children's performance out of categories that would indicate cause for concern in relation to speech and language development.

In the majority of the categories tested, the participants of the 'Speech Bubbles' groups made better progress than a 'control' group.

The comparatively better progress made by the children receiving the intervention in 2015–16 was found to be statistically significant in three out of six of the categories tested using the progression tool:

Understanding spoken language

Storytelling and narrative

Social interaction

(Price, 2016)

## Language and learning techniques for running a session

Basic principles for running speech, language and communication sessions and indeed teaching lessons can be vast.

This programme suggests using the following key strategies and techniques to engage children and to help children access the language and learning within sessions.

The principles are based on a mixture of theories and actual practice, including (but not exclusively) general SLCN practice, high-quality teaching expectations (SEN/DCOP Jan 2015) and the Learning Cycle (Kolb, 1984).

Key objectives for using these core techniques are as follows:

- The needs of ALL learners within groups can access language and learning

- We can ensure the best possible progress and outcomes for the students

- Practitioners are Developing and carrying out High Quality Teaching.

(SEN/D COP, Jan 2015)

### *The six principles are*

Recap/review

Memory and processing

Vocabulary

Expressive support

Story components

Levels of questioning

(This is described in more detail in a step-by-step format)

# (1) Recap and review

- Link with prior learning/lesson: intro to session should always include what happened last session / what they learned / links to this week's session.

- Provide opportunities to recap verbally – children to use their own words to recap last sessions or experiences or describe something they are learning that link with this week's story/session.

- Explicitly share links with learning: provide clear links to elsewhere in the curriculum or children's experiences where possible – e.g. 'Red Riding Hood' story: link to curriculum could be 'stranger danger' and how Red Riding Hood links with this or with their own experience; ask children, 'Have you ever been to visit someone who wasn't well or taken a nice present to someone?'

- Allow time for review of the session and learning at the end.

- Allow time throughout the session to recap and review what they are doing and how what they are doing links to the session's learning/targets.

# (2) Memory and processing

- Break instructions and language into manageable chunks.

- Repetition of instructions and language.

- Use of visual support – support spoken language through pictures/symbols/signs/props.

- Check that the child understands the task/activity.

- Allow time for children to process language and consider pace.

# (3) Vocabulary

- Repeat new or important vocabulary several times.

- Don't presume knowledge of vocabulary – check that children understand the words you are using – not just the target vocabulary in your session.

- When appropriate, use synonyms to help expand children's vocabulary: e.g. in the 'Hungry Caterpillar,' the practitioner explains he 'ate' through a green leaf . . . ask and give more words for ate: nibbled/chewed/munched/gobbled.

    There are parts within activities that specifically work on synonyms; however, look out for opportunities throughout the session to explore these where it is not mentioned.

- Use links with vocabulary to help children learn (where you find it / what it looks like / what it does / what its first sound is / clap out syllables).

## (4) Expressive support

- Provide sentence starters / question words to help children start their sentences or start their questions (can be verbal/written/symbol support)
- Give time for verbal planning and response.
- Opportunities for verbal rehearsal – paired talk, mixed ability, chants and repetitive lines.
- Model and extend child's verbalisations – e.g. modelling: child says, 'He readed the book!' And the practitioner models back, 'Yes! He read the book.' Practitioner could also suggest extending:

    Practitioner: 'Is it big or little?'

    Child: 'Big.'

    Practitioner: 'Yes! He read the big book!'

## (5) Story components

The sessions are based on story components and are used to scaffold children's storytelling.[7] Components are:

    Who

    Where

    When

What happened

The end

(A 'Problem' component is added at a later stage)

Children should be reminded of them at the beginning and at the end of the session by using examples from everyday life and the stories/topics they are learning.[8]

## (6) Levels of questioning

The levels of questioning technique is a key technique that can be used within this intervention programme during activities and at the end of sessions.

'Levels of questioning' were developed by Blank, Rose and Berlin (1978). The premise is that questions move from concrete to abstract. These questions can develop expressive skills and verbal reasoning.

The practitioners need to understand the complexity level of questions to help them simplify language or challenge language skills. Knowing these question levels helps the practitioner differentiate appropriately during the session and target particular levels of questions appropriately to children so that they are all challenged but also so that those at a lower level can feel success and have language aimed at their level.

Practitioners should think about the choice of questions in their planning of sessions and which questions they will direct at which children. These questions can also be used as a checklist to monitor where the children are and how they progress over time.

The levels are outlined below – examples are provided with the story 'Cinderella' as an example:

### Level one

Concrete thinking: questions relate to the immediate environment.

Examples include:

'What is that?' (Pumpkin)

'Find one like this.' (Glass slipper)

'What is Cinderella doing?' (Crying)

'Is it a castle? (Yes/no response)

## Level two

Involve some analysis such as grouping objects or describing and understanding object functions.

Examples include:

'Find something that can run' (Horse)

'What is happening in this picture?' (Cinderella is feeding the mice)

'Where is the mouse?' (Requires a location response – e.g. 'under the table' – not just pointing)

'Find something that is . . .' (E.g. 'orange and round': pumpkin)

'How are these different?' (This slipper is broken, and this slipper is not)

'Which one is . . . ?' (E.g. 'an animal': Dog)

## Level three

Children start using higher-order thinking. These questions ask the children to use their own knowledge to make basic predictions, assume the role of another, or make generalisations.

Examples include:

'What will happen next?' (Cinderella will not be able to go to the ball)

'How do you think she feels?' (Sad)

'How do I make . . . ?' (E.g. 'a dress': get some material, cut out a pattern, sew it together and stick on some sequins)

'How are these the same?' (They are both mean people)

'What is a . . . ?' (E.g. 'servant': someone who has to work and do jobs for another person)

## Level four

Involve problem solving, predictions, solutions and explanations. Require own knowledge and thinking about the future and past.

Examples include:

Predicting changes: 'What will happen if . . . [e.g. she doesn't hear the clock strike 12]?'

Solutions: 'What should she do now?'

Causes: 'How did that happen?'

Justifying: 'Why can't we . . . ?'

Explanations: 'How can we tell she is sad?'

## How to use

These questions can be asked after a story has been read, during a story, during the story square activity or during activities around a story: for example, playing a game where children are walking around the room acting out a character. . . . Practitioner asks one child, 'What are you doing?' (level one), and asks another child, 'What will you do if . . . ?' (level three).

# The drama part

Drama can be intimidating, and professionals often move away from it because of being overwhelmed by drama terminology and not wanting to get things wrong.

Often, therapists and teachers are unfamiliar with facilitating dramatic activities (Furman, 2000). Many feel intimidated by the idea of leading students in dramatic activities; however, most dramatic activities do not require practitioners to have direct theatre experience (Beehner, 1990).

It is worth remembering that this programme only uses drama techniques as a framework and that its main emphasis and technique is to make sessions interesting, fun and language enriched. They are to build on communication skills and not dramatic ability or an end performance.

The following information is to explain the majority (but not all) of the drama techniques this programme uses in simple terms.

## Process drama

- Includes all the drama techniques where adults and pupils work in-role

- Examples: Hot Seating, Teacher In-Role, Mantle of the Expert, Role-Play

- The drama happens within the context of a story

- Lead practitioners: Gavin Bolton, Dorothy Heathcote.[9]

Process drama is performed for the sake of the act of doing it. It is not for a final performance. It is not being made for an audience, and it doesn't need to be rehearsed.

The audience can be the children themselves. The important part of process drama is working through a problem and potentially seeing it from different perspectives.

The students 'engage in drama to make meaning *for themselves*' (Bowell and Heap, 2001).

Process drama is using dramatic forms with a group of children involved in the telling of a story. It can look at setting, text, dialogue, character, plot, climax, and beginning, middle and end of a story.

## Process drama techniques used in this programme

### Hot Seating

The group questions a character. This can be done where the hot seat has individuals, pairs or small groups sat on it. The practitioner is the facilitator and helps scaffold the questions and responses.

Some roles will require some setting up and knowledge from the practitioner . . . other characters may be already well known.

It would be good to encourage children to ask and answer about feelings and situations and what the character might do next – however, basic question asking may be the aim of the activity such as asking or understanding who/where/when/what questions.

Hot Seating can develop so that the person/people in the hot seat are in-role and the children asking questions are in-role. Props can also be used so that the children are in character when they are holding the prop and resume to themselves once not holding the prop.

## Mantle of the Expert

In a Mantle of the Expert,[10] a fictional world is created in which the children all have roles as an expert in a particular field. Their expertise can genuinely develop, and their understanding of certain concepts can be enhanced. Almost any area of the curriculum could be taught through a Mantle of the Expert.

Mantle of the Expert is based on the idea that children learn instinctively through imaginary play and that play is a generator of culture. Importantly, although play often matters to those involved, it carries no genuine penalty in the world of reality. It is a 'safe space' where children can explore ideas, events, people and narratives without ever having to be in any danger or having to cope with real consequences. (Taylor, 2016)

Examples can be pretending to be astronauts and preparing for a trip to space. . . . What will they need? What problems might occur? How will they communicate with earth? Or they could be zookeepers that need to rescue a visitor from a lion den. . . .

The children are not real experts and would never really fly into space or need to rescue someone from a lion. However, many would like to imagine themselves doing it, and this helps children become an active part of their learning and enables language and learning to be embedded at a deeper level.

In the normal practitioner-and-student relationship, the practitioner is usually 'the expert' and the children are the ones doing the learning. In Mantle of the Expert, the teacher deliberately plays around with roles of power and authority. When the children agree to take on the 'Mantle of the Expert,' they are the expert, and they can make choices and decisions and can change events. They also agree to take on the responsibilities, duties and roles of the expert team.

These scenarios can generate new language and can help children bring their narratives to life. They can also lead into other curriculum links such as letter-writing, designing a poster, links to geography and history, etc.

## Role-Play

Role-Play is the changing of behaviour to become another character.

Many children participate in a form of role-playing known as make believe or pretending . . . wherein they adopt certain roles such as doctor, mummy, superhero etc. and act out those roles in character.

Role-Play is the basis of all dramatic activity (Farmer, 2012).

## Forum theatre / image theatre

- This is developed from the practice and writings of Augusto Boal, a Brazilian theatre maker.[11]
- It uses theatre to explore solutions to a range of problems that arise through social inequality.
- Simplest form – making statues or images that bring physical form to problems, ideas and solutions.

## Forum/image theatre techniques used in this programme

### Forum

A scene is acted out and then repeated or 'replayed.' During the replay, any member of the group is allowed to shout 'Stop!' and take the place of one of the characters (usually the oppressed character: Cinderella / Sleeping Beauty). They then show how they could change the situation to enable a different outcome. This is good to use in the transition between imitating stories and beginning to change elements of stories to make them different.

### Freeze frames

With freeze frame, the action in a play or scene is frozen. This creates the effect of a photograph or video.

## Still images

This is when children create a scene or stories through still images (good for children who find the oral part of acting difficult).

## Thought tracking

Thought tracking can follow on from freeze frames and still images. Children within a freeze frame can be asked to speak the thoughts or feelings of their character aloud. This can start simply with one word and gradually expand.

Responses can be scaffolded by the practitioner's questions, such as 'What will they need to do next?'

## Story square

- Developed from 'Play What You Say' (by Vivian Gussin Paley, a kindergarten teacher in Chicago) and the Helicopter Technique (which grew out of Vivian Gussin Paley's book *The Boy Who Would Be a Helicopter*)
- Re-enacting stories in a story square
- Uses 'whoosh' technique by Dr Joe Winston.

'Play what you say' is a technique which involves children telling stories that are then scribed verbatim by an adult during private storytelling. Once the stories have been collected, a masking-tape square is marked on the floor, and these stories are then acted out and brought to life by the whole group.

This technique has now developed into being used with everyday stories and scenarios.

From a speech and language perspective, the children need their stories and narrative abilities developed, and they need tools, experience and scaffolding to enable this. Therefore, the story square practice has evolved so that it is not children's stories but any story that can be acted out within the square.

Once children's narratives and confidence improves, this technique can be implemented so that children's own stories are used in the square.

The story square enables the participants within it to be characters, objects, places and events. The children on the outside of the square can also be involved – for example, the practitioner says, 'There was a storm,' and the children around the circle can create the background noise of a storm.

Every child gets a turn, and the square is clearly marked out so that children know where to sit and the space size doesn't change.

## In summary

Drama techniques are not just fun and interesting ways to learn. As McMaster (1998) endorsed, drama can be an invaluable teaching method since it supports every aspect of literacy development.

From developing their decoding knowledge, fluency, vocabulary, syntactic knowledge, discourse knowledge and metacognitive knowledge to comprehension of extended texts, drama and theatre in many ways educate children as a whole, and they offer children a more free and flexible space in which to grow and learn.

## The story square

### *How to implement the 'story square'*

A square is marked out (usually with masking tape).

The whole group sits around the square. It is explained to the children that when the practitioner says 'Whoosh!' they should quickly return to the place they were sat. The 'Whoosh' technique was devised by Dr Joe Winston of the University of Warwick and first described in his 2008 book: *Beginning Drama 4–11*.

Once the story begins (read or told by the practitioner), the first character, event or object is mentioned, and the child chosen to start is prompted to step into the square to be that character or make a shape or pose. More than one character/object/event can be mentioned, and two to three children can stand and enter the square at the same time.

The practitioner should go around the square, and, as more characters and objects enter the story, more children can participate. Then if square gets too full or becomes a little too chaotic, or if it is the natural end of a scene, then the practitioner says

'Whoosh' (and uses a sweeping motion from left to right with his or her arm) and the children return to their place.

The children sat around the square can also be encouraged with eye contact and prompts to join in with shouting 'Whoosh' out loud and using the sweeping arm movement in time with the practitioner.

The square is then empty and ready to be filled again, and it also gives natural pause through the story.

The 'Whoosh' effect means that different children get to play the same and different characters and can try different roles and genders.

The children can interact with one another and express lines from the story.

## Example of story square activity

### 'Jack and the Beanstalk'

*Practitioner:* 'Once upon a time there was a boy named Jack.' (Point to first child and then prompt him or her to go into the square).

*Practitioner:* 'Jack lived with his mum and his cow called Daisy.' (Point to next child as practitioner says 'mum' and then point to next child as practitioner says 'cow.')

All three children are now in the square – child number 3 is maybe on all fours pretending to be a cow and saying 'Moo!'

*Practitioner:* 'Jack and his mum were very poor and hungry.' (*Children prompted to look hungry, sad, poor etc. – try prompting with just an expectant look so the flow can keep going, but children may need a verbal prompt at first – 'Can you all look hungry and sad?'*)

*Practitioner:* 'They lived in a very small crooked house.' (*Next child around the square pointed to so that he or she enters the square.*)

Child number 4 should now be making a house shape with his or her body – remind the child that it's *small* and *crooked* and explain 'crooked' if the child is unsure about the meaning.

| Practitioner: | 'Although she didn't want to, mum told Jack: "Take the cow to market and sell him!" ' (*Practitioner points to mum character who is in the square if the child needs prompt.*) |
| Mum character: | 'Take the cow to market and sell him!' |

Note: if the child has difficulty recalling words, split sentence in half: 'Take the cow to market' (child repeats this part) 'and sell him' (child repeats this part).

Practitioner:   'Jack was sad.' (Practitioner gives expectant look to child playing Jack.)

Jack character starts looking sad.

| Practitioner: | 'But Jack said to his cow: "Come on Daisy . . . let's go to market." ' |
| Jack character: | 'Come on Daisy . . . let's go to market.' |

Jack and cow character walk around square together pretending to be on way to market.

| Practitioner: | 'Whoosh.' |
| All children: | all children in square go back to their places. |
| Practitioner: | 'Whilst Jack (*point to next child around square, so he or she gets into square as Jack*) and Daisy (*point to next child so he or she gets into square as Daisy*) were on their way to market, they met an old man (*point to next child so that he or she gets into square as an old man – prompt child to think about how he or she can look old*).' |
| Practitioner: | 'The old man said to Jack: "Where are you going?" ' |
| Old man character: | 'Where are you going?' |
| Practitioner: | 'Jack replied: "I'm going to market to sell my cow." ' |
| Jack character: | 'I'm going to market to sell my cow.' |

The story progresses like this until eventually the magic beans are thrown out of the window (the window acted out by a child – possibly by the child making a big circle with his or her arms – but leave the child to use his or her imagination unless the child needs help) by Jack's mum. A child is then put into the square as the bean and slowly grows and grows as the practitioner (narrator) describes this:

| Practitioner: | 'The magic bean grew and grew and grew until it touched the sky . . . it was so tall!' |

The story then continues to progress . . .

## Benefits to speech, language and communication by using the story square

**Attention and listening:** the stories being re-enacted are very visual with children's peers acting inside the square. This helps children sustain attention due to high interest.

In addition children are actively anticipating when it is going to be their turn, and this encourages them to sustain their attention.

Children need to sustain attention during acting-out scenes, whether characters or objects. They are listening out for their part and what they need to do next.

**Vocabulary**: new vocabulary can be introduced and explored during story squares and can be put into context through the story – enabling children to link their new words with meaning and also experience them within acting to help embed new learning.

The story square will often focus on the adverbs and adjectives within a story so that children can express the character, object or event more accurately and so they take note of describing words:

E.g. how can they make a character look old, tired, sad, poor, magic, happy, suspicious etc.

Exposure to adjectives and adverbs in this way will help children develop vocabulary use and understanding.

**Expression**: children can practice lines from the stories and repeat verbatim what the characters say. This makes using language safe as they aren't generating it themselves, but at the same time they are reflecting on the words and structures of the sentences and applying them in context.

Repetition of language is an important skill to build on and is fundamental to language learning.

Children are encouraged to comment on the story and their favourite parts of the story square at the end – encouraging children to generate their thoughts and opinions through expressive language.

The story square models the structure of stories, providing a beginning, middle and end. The story square discussion is also facilitated by vital narrative elements, including: Who? Where? When? What? Ending?

These elements are repeated each session and provide a model and scaffold for children to start generating their own stories through a familiar framework and also encourage them to put more descriptive vocabulary within their stories.

**Understanding**: the story square is presented through auditory, visual and kinaesthetic mediums – all facilitating the child's understanding of the stories. The actual participation enables children to experience the stories and concepts.

The story square can help build inference, prediction and verbal reasoning skills.

Children have to listen to the story and understand what it is they should be acting out. The story square should be broken down to a word level the children understand so that all children can access the language and story. Word level and sentence length can then slowly be expanded to help the children's understanding and processing capacity develop (for instance, reducing language for children that need it – e.g. 'Jack got his cow . . . and walked to market').

**Pragmatics**: develops turn taking and makes turn taking visual to help children that find this difficult. The model is also familiar, and all children know the will get a turn, if not several turns, so they can anticipate that they will not be left out.

The story square develops children's skills for working together and group cohesiveness. It develops the understanding and use of facial expression, gesture and posture and develops confidence in using their bodies, expressing themselves and being within a group.

## Structure of sessions

These sessions take place within a basic format, consisting of four elements:

**(1) Introduction/review** – children sit around the story square and have an introduction to the session . . . what they are going to do . . . what they did last week and a recap on story components: who/where/when/what/ending?

The components can be about everyday life (e.g. 'Who did you walk to school with today? Where did you go for lunch today? When did you go on your school trip this week? What did you do after you got out of bed this morning? What will you do at the end of school today?').

Or

Linked to the story/topic children did last session (e.g. 'Who was in the story last week? Where was the story? When did the story happen? What happened? How did it end?').

Or

Linked to the story they are about to do . . . using prediction skills from being shown pictures of the book or any past experience with that story.

**(2) Warm up** – in preparation for the language and learning ahead.

This can be linked to the topic of that session – so that it presents as a pre-teaching format, but it can also just be a warm up where children re-familiarise themselves with the space, the context and each other.

They are characterised by games with low language load and aim to obtain and build on attention, listening and group cohesion.

**(3) Focus** – this is familiarising the children with the story/topic that the session is focusing on. This includes reading the story/topic and also engaging in activities, which are based around the story/topic.

**(4) Completion** – this marks the end of the main work and allows children time to reflect and review the language and learning within the session.

They also *de-roll* (leave their character) if they have been in character so that they leave the session as themselves. De-rolling can include 'shaking off' character by shaking limbs, giving props back, taking costume off or washing off character . . . children pretending to shower and 'washing off' the session.

*Moving on:*

The programme aims to work on familiar stories and stories/topics that are linked to the curriculum. Eventually, as children's skills progress, sessions can change so that they start to build on children's storytelling and creation of their own stories.

*Keeping control:*

Sessions like these can encourage excitement and sound levels that increase rapidly! It is important to remember that this is good at times and helps children feel relaxed and ready to communicate – however, establish group rules, and praise children who are displaying good group rules.

Have a signal, such as use of a tambourine or a clap pattern, to get children to stop their activity and refocus, and use this in all sessions.

*Timing:*

Sessions are designed to last around 45 minutes but can be made longer or shorter as appropriate.

## Evaluation and assessment

To summarise everything presented so far – here is the session model:

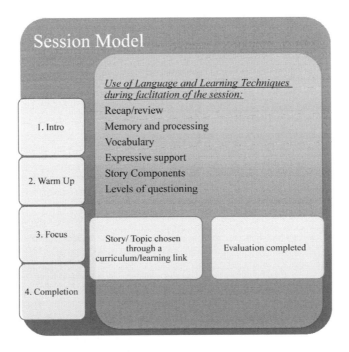

## *Evaluation*

Evaluation forms have been compiled so that sessions can be evaluated easily and quickly. The option of a single pupil evaluation can be used if a child-specific evaluation is needed, or a whole group evaluation can be used where evaluation focus is more on a group/session level.

Key Stage 1 and two examples are provided here . . . and other examples can be found in Appendix B alongside the evaluation sheets in Appendix A that can be copied and used by practitioners.

The single pupil evaluation forms can be used to monitor and compare progress from a child's first session to final session.

Evaluations are for practitioners to monitor what skills are being worked on in each session and any information they want to record to help plan future sessions. It is useful to keep records of sessions throughout the programme.

| Session Evaluation: Reception and Key Stage 1 | |
|---|---|
| **Session Number**: 3 **Story Session Title**: Funnybones Session One<br><br>**Pupils in Session**: Ellen, Anthony, Tammy, John, Gemma, Gregory, Elizabeth, Paul, Kate | |
| **Area of Speech, Language and Communication Targeted** | **Tick if Targeted** |
| **Non-verbal Skills:** | |
| Attention | ✓ |
| Listening | ✓ |
| Non-verbal communication / facial expression | ✓ |
| **Receptive Language Areas / Memory / Processing** | |
| Following instructions (within activity) | |
| Understanding question words . . . List question words targeted | |

| | |
|---|---|
| Understanding descriptions (e.g. following practitioner descriptions in activities)<br>Followed description for journey to story square | ✓ |
| Memory | |
| Processing | ✓ |
| **Expressive Language (Verbal)** | |
| Using complete sentences | ✓ |
| Using questions words . . . List question words targeted: | |
| Recalling sentences verbatim | ✓ |
| Sequencing | ✓ |
| **Phonological Awareness** | |
| Areas of phonological awareness worked on: | |
| **Higher-Level Language** | |
| Verbal reasoning | |
| Answering why / what if / how questions | |
| Prediction | ✓ |
| Inference | |
| **Narrative Skills** | |
| Understanding story in story square | ✓ |
| Story components covered in discussion: who, where, when, what, the end | ✓ |
| Contributing to story making | |
| Story components directly covered in activities: who, where, when, what, the end<br>No activities directly targeting these today | |
| **Vocabulary** | |
| Description vocabulary / concepts / feelings vocabulary within session:<br><br>Synonyms for frighten: petrified/scared/terrified/chilled<br><br>Actions you do if frightened: jump / shake / turn pale / go stiff / freeze | |

| | |
|---|---|
| Topic / story vocabulary targeted in session:<br><br>Bones<br>Skeletons<br>Dog<br>Body parts | |
| **Social Skills / Pragmatics** | |
| Turn taking | ✓ |
| Eye contact | ✓ |
| Conversation skills | |
| Social language (greetings, ending conversations etc.) | |
| Negotiation | |
| Tolerance | |
| Team work / cohesion | ✓ |
| **Areas Targeted Not Listed:** | |
| **Additional Comments/Notes:**<br>Funnybones session two next session<br>Anthony needs more work and feedback for attention and listening<br>Tammy very good at story components . . . doesn't need to answer these next week – focus more on Gregory and Ellen for these<br>Kate finds social skill activities difficult at times – joining in groups<br>Gemma takes lead in group work – separate her and Kate | |

Date:  30-09-17                    Signed: J Lea-Trowman

| Session Evaluation: Key Stage 2 | |
|---|---|
| **Session Number:** 4 | **Session Title:** Romans Session 4 |
| Pupils in Session: Carly, Amanda, Abbie, Zoe, Anna, Claire, | |

| Activity Delivered | SLCN Targeted |
|---|---|
| | Comments on Student Participation |

| Introduction: | |
|---|---|
| Recap on who: the different types of roman roles: emperor, slave, etc. . . . <br><br> Where: different places Romans used: baths, markets, homes, amphitheatres <br><br> When: recap on meaning of BCE and CE <br><br> What happened in story Romulus and Remus | Narrative elements to help recap: who, where, when, what happened? <br> Review and recap language from previous sessions <br> Sentences around the topic |
| | All named a Roman role or famous character <br> Abbie and Anna struggled with recall of BCE and CE <br> All retold elements of Romulus and Remus together |

| Warm Up: | |
|---|---|
| Months of the year line up <br><br> Carried out twice: (as 6 students) <br> Jan to June first time <br> July to Dec second time | Attention <br> Social skills: turn taking, collaboration, tolerance, patience, eye contact, non-verbal comm, group cohesion <br> Months of the year vocabulary and sequencing <br> 'when' component |
| | Zoe and Anna needed peer support with where to stand in months activity |

| Focus One: | |
|---|---|
| Roman towns | Attention and listening <br> Processing <br> 'Where' component <br> British places vocabulary <br><br><br> All enjoyed game – at the end each student could name one place that had Roman 'ending' |

| Focus Two: | |
|---|---|
| Hadrian's fact hunt | Attention and listening<br>Processing<br>Memory<br>Comprehension<br>Vocabulary<br>Social skills: turn taking, eye contact<br>Starting and finishing an interaction<br>'What' component |
| | had fact written down to aid memory. Others remembered facts.<br><br>Enjoyed mixing and social skills good<br><br>All could name one other fact at the end of activity – however Zoe needed some prompting from peer to remember length of wall. . . |

| **Completion:** | |
|---|---|
| Recap and shake off the session | De-roll |
| | All named a British place<br>Recited months of the year all together (to help support those who are still unsure)<br>All said their own Hadrian's Wall fact |

**Additional Comments:**

Do a BCE / CE activity next week to embed this further . . . another months of the year activity if possible – do timeline activity
Introduce Roman numerals, as covering this in class next week
Do another Hadrian's Wall activity to embed
Anna, Zoe and Abbie need more support
Carly needs some work on social skills
Claire reluctant to join in recap

Date: 20-02-17                    Signed: J Lea-Trowman

## Assessment

Assessment of a child's skills and progress can be formally analysed with Speech and Language Assessments carried out by a speech and language therapist.

Narrative assessments such as 'The Squirrel Story' and 'Peter and the Cat' (Black Sheep Press) are good pre- and post-measures to use as they can measure progress within a child's narrative skills.

This programme has an accompanying pre- and post-intervention assessment checklist.

The pre-intervention checklist can be completed before or during the first session. The practitioner can complete it in the session, or a teacher that knows the child well can complete it.

It is completed by answering whether each particular skill has been:

- Achieved (showing skill consistently and more than once)

- Partially achieved (showing skill occasionally but not always / skill is emerging)

- Not achieved (skill not seen / not emerging)

The checklist can then be completed again on the final session or around the final session, and scores can be compared to evaluate any change.

The scoring process is as follows:

- Achieved: scores 3

- Partially achieved: scores 2

- Not achieved: scores 1

The scores are then added together for a final score that is placed at the end of the assessment sheet. The two scores can be compared.

It is advised that the pre- and post-intervention markings are completed in different colours so it is clear which date is scoring what. The same person should complete the pre- and post-checklist.

An example of a checklist completed pre-/post-intervention follows.

| Name of Student: Nikki  Date Checklist Completed 1: 25-09-16  Date Checklist Completed 2: 15-05-17 | | | |
|---|---|---|---|
| | 1 | 2 | 3 |
| Area of Speech, Language and Communication | Not Achieved | Partially Achieved | Achieved |
| Attention (child able to attend for majority of activity) | | ✓ | ✓ |
| Listening (child showing listening skills in tasks) | | ✓✓ | |
| Non-verbal communication / facial expression (appropriate use of NV communication and facial expressions within activities requiring this) | | | ✓✓ |
| Following instructions (within an activity – not in general) | | ✓✓ | |
| Understanding story components / question words: | | | |
| Who: | | | ✓✓ |
| Where: | | ✓ | ✓ |
| When: | ✓ | ✓ | |
| What: | ✓ | | ✓ |
| The end: | | ✓ | ✓ |
| Understanding stories/descriptions (follows a story and can act out what he or she hears) | | ✓ | ✓ |
| Memory (can child remember simple words / sentences / responses of others) | | ✓✓ | |
| Child uses complete sentences | | ✓ | ✓ |
| Use of question words: is child able to ask questions starting with: | | | ✓✓ |
| Who | | | ✓✓ |
| Where | ✓ | ✓ | |
| When | | | ✓ |
| What | ✓ | ✓ | |
| How | | | |

| | | | |
|---|---|---|---|
| Can child recall most sentences verbatim | | ✓ | ✓ |
| Sequencing (can child sequence events in order) | | ✓ | ✓ |
| Rhyme (can child generate rhyming words) | | ✓ | ✓ |
| Initial sound (can child generate a word with a given initial sound) | ✓ | ✓ | |
| Can child answer higher-level questions: | ✓ | ✓ | |
| Why: | ✓✓ | | |
| What if: | ✓ | | |
| How questions: | | ✓ | |
| Prediction (can child make a prediction using language) | | ✓ | ✓ |
| Inference (can child make inferences from language: e.g. not be directly told but to infer from a description what is happening) | | ✓✓ | |
| Use of description vocabulary /concepts / feelings vocabulary: (does child use these consistently within descriptions) | | ✓ | ✓ |
| Turn taking (can child take turns appropriately) | | ✓ | ✓ |
| Eye contact (can child make eye contact appropriately) | | ✓✓ | |
| Conversation skills (can child engage in conversation with a peer) | ✓ | ✓ | |
| Social language (can child use greetings / enter conversations / end conversations appropriately) | ✓ | ✓ | |
| Negotiation (can child use persuasive language with peers) | ✓ | ✓ | |
| Tolerance / patience (can child wait for others appropriately) | | ✓ | ✓ |
| Team cohesion (can child work within a group appropriately) | | ✓ | ✓ |
| **Scores** | | | |
| **Total Assessment One:** | 11 | □□ | 1□ |
| **Total Assessment Two:** | 1 | □□ | □□ |

**Total Overall Assessment One =** 61

## Notes

1   Further reading: www.gov.uk/dfe/nationalcurriculum.

2   See http://www.foundationyears.org.uk.

3   For further reading and information: www.pshe-association.org.uk.

4   Available at http://www.londonbubble.org.uk/uploads/SO_Evaluation_5371.pdf.

5   Please see: 'Speech Bubbles' Drama Intervention Programme Preliminary Executive Summary of Effectiveness (Dr Heather Price, Psychological Studies Research Group, School of Social Sciences, UEL).

6   Available at https://www.thecommunicationtrust.org.uk/resources/resources/resources-for-practitioners/progression-tools-primary/.

7   See Black Sheep Press for a version of narrative components www.blacksheeppress.co.uk.

8   See Appendix E for story component symbols that can be used in sessions.

9   For further reading, see: Drama for Learning: Dorothy Heathcote's Mantle of the Expert Approach to Education Dorothy Heathcote, Gavin M. Bolton, Pearson Education 1995.

10  For further information: www.mantleoftheexpert.com.

11  For further reading: *Theatre of the Oppressed*: Augusto Boal, Pluto Press, 1979.

# Chapter two
# THE PRACTICE

## Warm ups

These are general warm-up games mainly for working on bringing the group together and for children to focus and start using their bodies and getting their voices ready for this session.

A warm up should always be included in the structure of the session for this purpose but also as a routine for the participants.

Some session plans will contain theme-related/story-related warm ups already. Those that do not will reference 'See Warm Up Activities,' meaning that any of the following warm-up games can be chosen and carried out for that session. These warm ups can also be used at the beginning of other therapy sessions/lessons!

### Group counting

The group stands in a circle. The group must count from 1 to however many people are in the circle. Only one person at a time may speak, and the counting shouldn't go in order round the circle. Once someone has said a number, that person should sit down. If two people speak at once, everyone stands up again and the count goes back to 1.

If the group manages this, the exercise can be repeated with everyone standing up again once they've said a number (this way round is easier).

Developing: Eye contact / turn taking / group cohesion / attention and listening skills

### Ten Seconds to . . .

Everyone in the room has ten seconds to . . .

Shake as many hands as possible

Shake feet with as many people as possible

Tap everyone on the shoulder

Touch all four walls

Introduce yourself to people in the style of the queen

Slap everyone around the face with an imaginary wet fish

Apologise!

Get into a perfect circle.

> Developing: Eye contact / turn taking / group cohesion / non-verbal communication / attention and listening skills

## Object game

Get the group to form a circle. Place an everyday object in the centre of the circle. One at a time volunteers come forward and use the object for something else entirely, either using mime, sound or speech.

Then ask individuals to 'freeze' mid-scene, and get another volunteer to join them in the centre of the circle and continue the scene together.

> Developing: Eye contact / turn taking / non-verbal communication / tolerance of a peer / attention and listening skills

## Jump stop, clap, go!

This is a great activity for developing the group as an ensemble and for developing listening and concentration skills. Participants walk around the space. They should be aware of where others are around them and try to fill all the space in the room. The leader then introduces two commands. Jump stop. Once they are following this, introduce two more: clap and go.

Once the group has got the hang of the commands, reverse them (i.e. 'stop' means 'go,' 'clap' means 'jump' etc.). This may need a slow build up – so only change to the opposites for two actions to start with.

Developing: Attention and listening skills / processing skills / space awareness

## Traffic lights

Children walk around the room finding space. Practitioner shouts out a traffic-light colour, and children do the following

Red – freeze

Amber – stand on one leg

Green – Go.

Practitioner can speed instructions up to make it more difficult – children can be 'out' if last and sit down – making obstacles for those left to walk around.

Developing: Attention and listening

## Slow-motion race

Participants are asked to 'race' from one end of the room to the other. However, the race must be done in slow motion. Whoever can move the slowest is the winner!

Developing: Awareness of others / attention

## Pass a clap

(1) Participants stand in a circle.
(2) The leader passes a clap around the circle (everyone claps one at a time until it gets back to the leader).
(3) Challenge the group to see how fast they can go, and time it.
(4) Change so they pass the clap across the circle to someone else – using eye contact and direction of clap to engage the other person.

Developing: Eye contact / turn taking / group cohesion / attention

### Hi!

Children stand in a circle. One child begins the game by pointing directly at someone across the circle from them and shouts 'Hi' in an aggressive way. The child then marches directly towards that person and takes that person's space in the circle. The person who's been pointed to moves the 'Hi' on to someone else. This continues. Extension: change the nature of the 'Hi' – it could be a sad 'Hi,' or a creepy 'Hi,' or a caring 'Hi' . . . etc.

> Developing: Eye contact / turn taking / attention / adverb understanding and expression

## Balloon pass

Children stand in a circle. One child begins the game by holding the balloon and carrying it across the circle to someone and then hands it to him or her – taking his or her space. That person then crosses the circle to pass the balloon to another person – making eye contact as he or she crosses.

Extension: the person carrying the balloon can say the other person's name while walking towards him or her and extend further naming of themselves: e.g. 'Edward to Aryton.'

> Developing: Eye contact / turn taking / attention skills

## Balloon pat

Children stand in a circle. One child begins the game by standing in the centre of the circle and throws the balloon up in the air. That person shouts another child's name (e.g. 'Sam'), and then Sam runs into the middle of the circle and pats the balloon up as he shouts another child's name, 'Rae,' who runs in, and so on. The aim is to make sure the balloon doesn't touch the floor, and that everyone's name around the circle is called.

> Developing: Turn taking / attention and listening / group cohesion

## Name in the bucket

Get the group to form a circle. Practitioner carries over an imaginary bucket and places it in the middle of the circle. All children have to 'throw' their names into the bucket by saying their names and using their hands to pretend to throw.

The children are encouraged to say their names in an unusual way . . . e.g. elongate it, use a squeaky voice, use a low voice, speak quickly, speak slowly etc.

Extend: discuss how the child said his or her name – attaching a describing word to it . . . e.g. Charlie said his name 'slowly' – or ask children to describe how the child said his or her name.

Developing: Turn taking / describing vocabulary / attention / using voice patterns

## Name catch

Children sit in a circle, and one child holds the ball. Make sure everyone is paying attention and making eye contact. . . . Emphasise importance of eye contact in this part of the game. The child says his or her name and rolls the ball to another child. That child then says his or her own name and rolls to someone else.

Extend by then getting the child with the ball to say his or her own name and the name of the person he or she is rolling to: 'Woody to Olivia.'

Extend again by asking another child, 'Who rolled to whom?'

'Archie . . . who had the ball in that sequence?'

This could start with two but then build up – e.g. Archie: 'Woody to Olivia, and Olivia to Rudy.'

Developing: Eye contact / turn taking / attention skills / memory / group cohesion

## Alliteration names

Children stand in a circle, and when it is their turn they do an action or give a describing word, which starts with the same letter as the first letter of their name . . . they say the words and do the action/description, and then everyone in the circle copies.

For example: 'Jumping Josie!' – Josie says this and jumps . . . then everyone in the circle together, facilitated by practitioner, jumps and says in unison, 'Jumping Josie!' Other examples: 'Star-jump Starla,' 'Pirouetting Poppy,' 'Laughing Lara-May,' 'Rolling Rafferty,' 'Moody Marley,' 'Eating Eva-Betsy,' 'Sly Sunny,' 'Fabulous Fran,' 'Tired Tammy,' 'Icy Isla' . . .

If a child finds the describing word too tricky to think of, then the practitioner can give them a word to use.

Developing: Eye contact / turn taking / attention and listening skills / phonological awareness (alliteration / initial sound) / describing vocabulary / verbs

## I can make a sound like this . . .

Children sit or stand in a circle, and practitioner starts by saying, 'I can make a sound like this: ahhh . . . ahhhhhhhhhh . . . ahhh.' Then everyone copies that sound all together in unison: 'ahhh . . . ahhhhhhhhhh . . . ahhh.'

The next chid in the circle then says the same sentence starter with a different sound: 'I can make a sound like this: eeeeeeee,' and everyone together copies 'eeeeeeee.'

Sounds can be with the mouth or with the body – e.g. thumping chest . . . clapping hands . . . slapping thighs . . . . tapping the floor . . . stamping feet . . . etc.

Developing: Turn taking / attention and listening skills / imitation / use of voice patterns

## Different greetings

Children walk around the room . . . and then practitioner says, 'Freeze.' When they stop, they have to find a partner near them to say hello to. Once the children are paired up, the practitioner shouts out the context in which they must say hello . . . e.g.:

Pretend you haven't seen them for a very long time

Say hello as though you have just been for a run

Say hello like you are an alien

Pretend you are on the moon

Say hello like you have never met

Pretend you are under water

Pretend you have just woken up. . . .

> Developing: Eye contact / turn taking / attention and listening / non-verbal communication / role-play

## What are you doing?

Stand in a circle. The first child (e.g. Alice) starts acting out an activity – e.g. hanging out the washing – and the person next to Alice (e.g. Oliver) says, 'What are you doing?' Alice keeps acting out the activity (hanging out the washing) but says a different activity – e.g. 'playing football.' Oliver then starts acting out playing football, and Alice sits down. The next child in the circle (e.g. Elodie) says to Oliver, 'What are you doing?' Oliver acts out football but says, 'Disco dancing.' Elodie then starts to disco dance, and Oliver sits down . . . then the next child asks Elodie, 'What are you doing?' and so on . . .

> Developing: Eye contact / turn taking / attention and listening / non-verbal communication / verb vocabulary / social skills (entering an activity)

## Vocabulary ball roll

Children sit in a circle and roll the ball to someone across the circle. They are given a category in which they name vocabulary from. The child must label a vocabulary item as he or she rolls the ball: e.g. fruits, animals, transport etc.

Current class topics could be used for the story of the session– e.g. Rumpelstiltskin: baby / princess / name / straw / gold

Rumpelstiltskin / woods / promise / prince . . .

Developing: Eye contact / turn taking / attention and listening / vocabulary / categorising

## What's different?

Children sit in a circle, and then two children get in the middle, sitting opposite each other. One child then turns around so the child can't see his or her partner, and the partner changes something about his or her own appearance (takes a shoe off, unbuttons a button, twists a tie, takes out a hair clip, etc.).

The partner then turns back around and has to say what has changed: 'Eddie has taken out her hair clip.'

Extension: increase the number of things the partner changes.

Developing: Eye contact / attention / visual memory / sentence completion

## Group rules

Children should be explicitly taken through the rules of the session during the introduction so they know expectations and so these skills can be commented on and developed.

Visuals can accompany the rules:

Taking turns

Looking at each other or the person when talking

Listening to each other

Being kind to each other and respect each other's contributions

Sitting around the story square.

# The Very Hungry Caterpillar
By Eric Carle

## Curriculum links

- SEAL – changes / healthy Eating

- Science – life cycles / growing

- Geography – different environments

- Maths – days of the week / adding / subtracting

- Narrative unit – story with familiar setting

- Topics  mini-beasts / growth and change / in the garden

## *Session 1*

## Introduction

*Sit around the story square.*

Recap on group rules:

Introduce 'The Very Hungry Caterpillar' book briefly with story components (who, where, when, what, the end) to support.

*Who* – caterpillar

*Where* – garden

*When* – day and night / days of week / discuss how caterpillars on average stay in cocoon for two weeks

*What* – caterpillars eat and then make a cocoon to help them transform

Developing:
- Understanding group rules
- Understanding of story components
- Understanding story
- Story familiarity

*The end* – into a butterfly

Describe how session will run and content of session.

Read the book: 'The Very Hungry Caterpillar.'

## Warm up

### Discrimination walk

Children walk around the room. . . . Different items from the book are said out loud by practitioner, and children listen for them . . .

If they hear an item that isn't in the book, they should get down to the floor and curl up in a cocoon.

Developing:
- Attention and listening
- Vocabulary categorisation/discrimination
- Exposure to book vocabulary

## Focus 1

### Cocoons

Get everyone to find a space and curl up into a cocoon.

Discuss: What is a cocoon?

The caterpillar feels warm inside. . . . Can children generate other words for 'warm'? For example: cosy, snuggly, toasty etc.

Developing:
- Attention
- Vocabulary extension with synonyms
- Vocabulary from book
- 'Who' component

Discuss the concept/word 'turn into.'

Can children generate other words for 'turned into'? For example: change, transform, metamorphosis, evolve, mutate, alter.

Children to slowly break out of their cocoons and become butterflies . . . listening to the different words for 'turned into' being used by practitioner as they grow and become butterflies.

Children then flap arms and fly around the room filling the space . . .

Ask children to stop flying. . . . Can any of them remember any of the new words they heard for 'turn into'?

Emphasise the word 'who' with story component card. . . . Who were they, and who have they turned into?

## Focus 2

### Group object

All children are to find a space in the room, and then ask them to make shapes of the fruit in the book (plum is oval, strawberry is heart shape, apple is round etc.). Encourage them to think how their bodies can make these fruits.

Progress onto children then getting into small groups.

They are given an item out of the book to recreate as a group: leaf, caterpillar, cake, lollipop, pickle, watermelon slice, ice cream . . . etc.

Developing:
- Attention
- Vocabulary extension
- Social skills: Group cohesion/ negotiation/ turn taking
- 'What' component

The groups are given time to recreate the shape and work together, and then groups show each other their creations. The other groups watching have to guess what items they are.

## Completion

### Sit around story square.

Recap and review:

Go through story components linked to 'The Very Hungry Caterpillar':

Who – caterpillar

Where – on a leaf / in the garden / into the sky

Developing:
- Story Component understanding
- Expressive and Receptive language skills around the story

When – night with egg, and day with caterpillar, also days of the week

What happened – egg hatched / caterpillar ate and ate / made a cocoon

The end – turned into a butterfly.

Everyone have a pretend shower: wash off the session and de-roll.

## Session 2

### Introduction

*Sit around the story square.*

Recap on group rules:

Children to answer story component questions related to the book (who, where, when, what, the end).

Describe how session will run and content of session.

Developing:

- Understanding group rules
- Understanding of story components
- Understanding story
- Story familiarity

### Warm up

*Days-of-the-week march*

The practitioner stands at one end of the room, and all children stand in a line next to the practitioner with backs against the wall. The practitioner then starts marching forwards while saying the days of the week – encourage the children to join in.

Developing:

- Attention and Listening
- Group cohesion/ awareness
- 'When' component
- Days of the week

The children have to march and stay in line with the practitioner.

The practitioner will shout 'stop' at some point and stop marching immediately . . . the children have to try to stop with the practitioner. Those children that step forwards and are out of line have to go back to the wall and march from there. . . . This repeats until some children get to the other side of the room with the practitioner.

Emphasise the word 'when' with the story component card . . . explain that the days of the week are used in story and that this is 'when' the caterpillar ate different foods.

## Focus 1

### *Butterflies*

Children fly around the room like butterflies – they must fly reflecting the word they are given:

Fly like you are angry/sad/excited/confused/happy/tired/etc.

Extend this to children being given a location and flying like they are in particular environments:

Fly like you are in a dark cave / hurricane / busy shopping centre / rainy mountain / sunny garden / snowy mountain . . .

Emphasise the word 'where' with the story component card . . . and link to different locations.

Developing:
- Attention and Listening
- Emotion vocabulary understanding
- 'Where' component understanding

## Focus 2

### *Story square*

Acting out the book of the hungry caterpillar. . . . Children can be caterpillar / moon / food items / butterfly / sun.

For example:

'In the light of the moon (*practitioner guides child to be moon*) an egg (*practitioner guides child to be egg*) lay on leaf. . . .'

'The sun came up (*practitioner guides child to be sun*) and egg turns into caterpillar.'

Developing:
- Attention and Listening
- Story understanding
- Narrative development
- Processing
- Social Skills (eye contact/ sharing space & cooperation/
- Non-Verbal communication (NVC)

'WHOOSH . . .'

Children then come into the square and become fruits. . . . Encourage them to be the shape.

'On Friday, he ate through five oranges' (*five children guided to come into story square to be oranges*) . . .

## Completion

### Sit around story square.

Recap and review:

> Go through story components linked to 'The Very Hungry Caterpillar.'

Everyone have a pretend shower: wash off the session and de-roll.

## Additional activities or alternatives

### Caterpillar footsteps

Quickly generate names of different mini-beasts: spider, worm, ant, fly, centipede etc. . . . You may need some visuals for this to help the child that will be labelling.

Play a game similar to Grandma's footsteps . . .

A child turns his or her back to other children (the child is the leader), and other children are on the other side of the room.

Developing:
- Story Component understanding
- Expressive and Receptive language skills around the story

Developing:
- Attention and Listening
- Vocabulary categorising

The leader will shout out a mini-beast – if the other children are sure that it is a mini-beast, they step forwards closer to the leader. If the child shouts out something that isn't a mini-beast, the children can all run away and the leader can turn and run to catch another child.

*This can also be done with healthy and non-healthy food categories.

## What happened next?

Use story cards to prompt and develop narrative. What happened after the book finishes?

Encourage connectives between each segment: so / and / because / then / next / after.

Encourage addition of describing words.

Developing:
- Attention and listening
- Narrative development
- Story components/ story language
- Sequencing
- Use of connectives
- Describing vocabulary

- When did the butterfly fly away? (can also use story language: once upon a time / after a while)

- Where did the butterfly fly to?

- Who did the butterfly meet?

- What did they do?

- The end?

Example story: 'After a while, the beautiful butterfly flew to a park and found some friends. She met a big spider and a spotty ladybird. They all played on the roundabout and got dizzy and then went to the colourful flowers for a long sleep because they were so tired!'

## The Rainbow Fish

By Marcus Pfister

### Curriculum links

- SEAL – getting on and falling out / friendship and sharing

- Narrative unit – stories in familiar settings

- Science – materials: shiny and dull

- Geography – different environments / habitats

- Maths – subtracting

- Topics – under the sea

## *Session 1*

### Introduction

*Sit around the story square.*

Recap on group rules:

Go over story component cards about general things: who, where, when, what, the end.

Introduce 'The Rainbow Fish' book (no need to read – just summarise).

Describe how session will run and content of session.

> Developing:
> - Understanding group rules
> - Understanding of story components
> - Understanding story
> - Story familiarity

### Warm up

*Pass the scale*

Warm-up activity same as 'balloon pass' from warm-up section of this book – however, to link to this story theme, cut out a large scale from foil or shiny material and use this instead.

> Developing:
> - Eye contact
> - Turn taking
> - Attention skills
> - Story vocabulary

### Focus 1

*Sea creatures*

Spread out around the room – generate in a group lots of animals that live under the sea . . .

When a child thinks of one – everyone move around the room like 'this' ('this' can be the practitioner modelling the movement or the child themselves if they feel confident to generate).

For example: octopus wavy arms, fish flapping with mouth opening and

> Developing:
> - Attention
> - Social skills: eye contact/turn taking
> - Playground rehearsal language
> - Vocabulary – ocean
> - Expression around feelings
> - 'Who' story component

closing, star fish jumping around in a star shape, dolphin swimming and jumping, shark with hand as its fin and making sharp movements etc. . . .

Ask children to then choose a creature/animal that lives under the sea and move around the room like it.

Encourage them to try to be different from others in the group.

One child is chosen to be 'the rainbow fish' and swims round the room . . . when that child come across another child, the first child needs to ask, 'Can I play with you?' The other child has to answer either yes or no . . . if the other child says yes, he or she goes behind the fish and goes with the fish to ask another child if he or she can play . . . if the new child says no, they carry on moving around the room as the creature they have chosen.

Once the activity is finished, everyone sit around the story square. . . . Ask the children how do they think the fish felt when another sea creature said they wouldn't play with them? How did the fish feel when other sea creatures said they would play with them?

Extend by asking the sea creatures how did they feel saying yes/no?

Emphasise the word 'who' with the story component card. . . . Who were they?

## Focus 2

### Story square

Acting out the book of 'The Rainbow Fish' . . .

This story has speaking parts so children can copy the lines from the book as they are read and prompted through the practitioner.

For example: one child in square as the rainbow fish swimming . . .

Developing:

- Attention and Listening
- Story understanding
- Narrative development
- Processing
- Sequencing
- Spoken language recall
- Social Skills: eye contact/ sharing space & cooperation
- Non-Verbal communication.

The little fish (prompt a child to come into square) said, 'Rainbow Fish wait for me. . . .'

'You want my scales?' said the Rainbow Fish. . . .

'WHOOSH . . .'

The story progresses with other characters . . . get to the part of 'now he was the loneliest fish.'

(Encourage child to look sad and lonely.)

Towards the end, select more than one child to be several fish calling over to the Rainbow Fish.

## Completion

*Sit around story square.*

Recap and review:

> Story components linked to 'The Rainbow Fish':
>
> Who: rainbow fish / little fish / starfish / octopus
>
> Where: ocean / dark cave
>
> When: day and night
>
> What happened: Rainbow Fish had beautiful scales / wanted friends but wouldn't give scales away / met with the octopus who gave him advice / Rainbow Fish gave scales away to others
>
> The end: the little fish all became friends with the Rainbow Fish, and now he only had one shiny scale . . .

Developing:
- Story Component understanding
- Expressive and Receptive language skills around the story

Discuss sharing and how it can be difficult to share – why did Rainbow Fish find it difficult to share?

Everyone have a pretend shower: wash off the session and de-roll.

## Additional activities or alternatives

### *Hot seat*

Discuss together what 'advice' means.

One child is chosen to be the octopus and sits in a chair or sits pretending he or she is in his or her cave.

Other children take turns to sit in front of octopus with a problem – the child needs to think of a problem.

Practice a sentence starter all together: 'My problem is that . . .' The octopus then gives them some advice.

The practitioner should model a turn first: 'My problem is . . . that I can't find my keys to the house!'

Octopus is given a sentence starter for each turn: 'My advice is . . .'

The octopus role can change so that other children get a turn in this more challenging roll.

Developing:
- Expressive language
- Understanding
- Verbal reasoning
- Problem solving
- Turn taking

# Room on the Broom

By Julia Donaldson

**Curriculum links**

- SEAL – relationships / friendship

- Narrative unit – predictable and patterned language / stories from the same author

- Science – weather

- Geography – different environments

- Topics – Halloween / adventures and fantasy

## Session 1

### Introduction

*Sit around the story square.*

Recap on group rules:

Go over story component cards about general things: who, where, when, what, the end.

Introduce 'Room on the Broom' book.

(No need to read – just summarise.)

Discuss what children already know about witches / the book.

Describe how session will run and content of session.

> Developing:
> * Understanding group rules
> * Understanding of story components
> * Familiarity of story
> * Story familiarity

### Warm up

*Name in the cauldron*

Same activity as 'name in the bucket' from the warm-up section . . . change *bucket* to a *cauldron* to match theme.

### Focus one

*Character crossover*

Children line up opposite each other (e.g. if ten in group, then five on each side).

The practitioner introduces the character 'who' (witch / cat / dog / bird / frog / dragon) – everyone discuss the character and how they may present (dog: tongue out panting / wagging tail / barking / happy . . . dragon: big / fierce / breathing fire . . . etc.)

> Developing:
> * Attention
> * Vocabulary extension
> * 'Who' component
> * Social skills; eye contact/ Non verbal communication

Then when the practitioner says go, the children walk towards each other and then past each other as that character so they have 'crossed over.'

Children then turn around and face each other again and then discuss the next character and cross over again as that character and so on. . . .

## Focus 2

### *Soundscape*

Children discuss where the witch flies: river / mountain / forest / bog.

For example: forest: wind in trees / snapping twigs / birds / trampling leaves / etc.

Developing:
- Attention and listening
- Vocabulary extension
- 'Where' component

One child then leaves briefly, and the group is given a place to re-create. Each child makes a different sound so the sounds all come together for the re-creation.

The child comes back in and listens to the group and guesses where they are.

## Completion

### *Sit around story square.*

Recap and review:

Story components linked to 'Room on the Broom.'

Everyone have a pretend shower: wash off the session and de-roll.

Developing:
- Story component understanding
- Expressive and receptive language skills around story

## Session 2

### Introduction

### *Sit around the story square.*

Recap on group rules:

Go over story component cards about 'Room on the Broom': who, where, when, what, the end.

Describe how session will run and content of session.

Developing:
- Understanding group rules
- Understanding of story components
- Familiarity of story

## Warm up

Choose a warm-up game from those provided in warm-up section. . . .

## Focus 1

### *Story square*

Acting out the book of 'Room on the Broom' . . .

This story has speaking parts so children can copy the lines from the book as they are read and prompted through the practitioner.

Encourage children who are not in the square to recreate the sounds of the scene being acted out . . . this has been rehearsed previously in soundscape activity.

Developing:

- Attention and Listening
- Story understanding
- Narrative development
- Processing
- Sequencing
- Spoken language recall
- Social Skills: eye contact/ sharing space & cooperation
- Non-Verbal communication.

## Focus 2

### *Freeze frame*

Children split into small groups.

Each group is given a scene to re-create as a still frame. The children must work together to create this. Once they have it rehearsed and ready, the groups show each other their freeze frames, and the other group/groups have to guess which scene they have re-created.

An extension to this is the practitioner taps a child on the shoulder, and the child shouts out a line from the book that his or her character says, or the child makes something up that his or her character might say.

Developing:

- Attention
- Social skills. Group cohesion/ negotiation
- Expressive and receptive language skill development in peer context
- 'What' component

## Completion

### Sit around story square.

Recap and review:

> Use levels of questioning.
>
> Discuss how kind the witch is and how she shares – can each child think of something they have shared before?

Developing:
- Story component understanding
- Expressive and receptive language skills around story

Everyone have a pretend shower: wash off the session and de-roll.

## Additional activities or alternatives

### Pass the hat

One child comes out of the square and faces away from the other children – the other children then pass a hat (a witch's preferably) around the square to each other.

Developing:
- Attention
- Vocabulary generation and categorisation

When the child standing says 'stop,' the child holding the hat puts the hat on and says a word linked to 'witch' (black / hat / pointy nose / broom / cat / cackle / Halloween / dress / cauldron / spooky / etc.).

The practitioner can change the vocabulary generation to children naming a story: with a witch in (Wizard of Oz / Sleeping Beauty / Snow White / Brave / Rapunzel / Winnie the Witch / Meg and Mog / etc.) or vocabulary linked to the dragon, etc.

### What next . . .

Children discuss with the practitioner what might happen next after the story has finished . . . where will they go on their new broom?

Developing:
- 'The end' component
- 'What' component
- Narrative development
- Prediction and inference skills
- Story generation
- Story square skills

Make a scenario up together with some dialogue and act out in the story square.

## The Shopping Basket

By John Burningham

### Curriculum links

- SEAL – no to bullying / relationships

- Narrative unit – stories with familiar settings

- Maths – counting and subtraction

- Topics – animals / shopping

### *Session 1: language and story focus*

## Introduction

*Sit around the story square.*

Recap on group rules:

Describe how session will run and content of session.

Go through story components linked to shopping: who do children go shopping with? Where do they go? When? What do they buy? What happens at the end of a shop?

Read story: 'The Shopping Basket.'

Developing:
- Understanding group rules
- Familiarity of story
- Story component understanding and expression

## Warm up

Choose a warm-up game from those provided in the warm-up section. . . .

## Focus 1

*Character game*

The children name four or five characters from the book. The practitioner asks a child how the animal might move or what the animal says.

The children are to walk around the room, and the practitioner shouts out a character . . . the children then move round the room like this and say the line from the book linked to that character. They repeat this until another character is shouted out.

Developing:
- Attention and listening
- Describing vocabulary
- Expressive language recall and rehearsal
- 'Who' component

For example:

Steven: walking around pretending to hold a basket saying: 'You are so slow I bet you couldn't even catch it.'

Bear: children stomping round trying to be big and heavy, saying: 'I will hug all the breath out of you.'

Monkey: children acting out a monkey with bodies saying, 'Give me those bananas or I'll pull your hair.'

Kangaroo: children jumping round the room saying, 'I'll punch you!'

## Focus 2

### Food numbers

Children walk around the room. When the practitioner shouts 'stop,' everyone stops . . . the practitioner will then shout out food and number so the children have to get themselves into groups of that number – for example: 'four apples' or 'five bananas.'

Try to use numbers so that no one is left out or, if someone is left over, the child can take a turn in shouting out the food and number on the next turn.

Extend: the children stand in their groups, and the practitioner asks everyone to count the number of children. Then take a child away and ask everyone, 'How many are left?'

Developing:
- Attention and listening
- Social skills; eye contact/ group cohesion
- Processing
- Counting
- Maths language

Use different words for 'take away' each time, and explain to the children that these words mean the same thing in a math problem: take away / subtract / minus.

## Focus 3

### Story square

Acting out the book of 'The Shopping Basket' . . .

This story has speaking parts, so children can copy the lines from the book as they are read and prompted through the practitioner.

Remember that children can also be objects such as a door, railings, a litter basket, etc.

Developing:

- Attention and Listening
- Story understanding
- Narrative development
- Processing
- Sequencing
- Spoken language recall
- Social Skills: eye contact/ sharing space & cooperation
- Non-Verbal communication.

## Completion

### Sit around story square.

Recap and review:

Story components linked to 'The Shopping Basket' (who, where, when, what, the end).

Ask children what their favourite thing was about what the child that sat next to them did.

Developing:

- Story component understanding
- Expressive and receptive language skills around story
- Awareness of others/ feedback language

Everyone shakes off the session: de-roll.

## Additional activities or alternatives

### Story path

The children are to create a path similar to the one in the story. One child is a door / another child is the railings / another is a litter basket / another is digging up pavement / and another child is the house where the dog lived.

This is stretched across the room, and then each remaining child 'walks the path' past the different locations.

The practitioner emphasises the 'where' element in this section.

> Developing:
> - Working with others
> - Social skills/ eye contact
> - 'Where' component

As a child gets to each location, the child can choose to walk down the path going past all the children to the other end or to stop at one of them and join that person in making the shape of the location object (e.g. join the railings person and hold his or her hand to make railings longer etc.).

At the end, when all children have walked the path, ask each child, ' "Where" did you stop?' etc. . . . .

## Session 2: bullying focus

## Introduction

### Sit around the story square.

Recap on group rules:

Describe how session will run and content of session.

Go through story components linked to 'The Shopping Basket' story.

> Developing:
> - Understanding group rules
> - Familiarity of story
> - Language analysis
> - Exploring word 'bullying'

Discuss bullying and how the characters show bullying behaviour and language in the book (e.g. kangaroo says, 'Or I'll thump you' – which word is unkind or bullying language?).

## Warm up

Choose a warm-up game from those provided in warm-up section. . . .

## Focus one

### Bully or victim?

Discuss bullies and victims . . . what these words mean. . . . How might bullies behave (hit / mean / pull faces / shout / push / angry)? How might the bullied person behave/ feel (sad / cry / scared / hide / run away / etc.)?

Children stand in a circle facing inwards. A child comes into the middle and does a freeze frame as either a bully or a victim (e.g. crouched down hiding / holding up fists / crying / scared / angry / pushing), and the other children say whether the person in the middle is pretending to be a bully or a victim.

Developing:
- Attention
- Vocabulary around bullying/emotions
- Answering 'why' questions/higher level thinking

Practitioner emphasises and narrates what the child is showing: e.g. 'Henry is showing an angry face, and his body looks stiff and threatening.'

## Focus two

### *Bully freeze frame*

Children are in pairs. They are asked to freeze frame an image of two people playing together. Tap on their shoulders.

When they are tapped on shoulder, they should try to explain how the children in their freeze frame that they are acting out feel.

Developing:
- Attention
- Social skills: eye contact / conversation skills
- Receptive and expressive language
- Prediction and inference

Children are then asked to freeze frame a situation where one person is being bullied.

Tap on shoulder.

Ask them to explain how they feel and what might happen next.

## Completion

### *Sit around story square.*

Recap and review:

Ask each child something about bullying that he or she can tell everyone (e.g. you can tell a teacher, bullying makes people sad . . . etc.).

Developing:
- Sentence construction
- Use of language learned and rehearsed in sessions

Everyone have a pretend shower: wash off the session and de-roll.

# Owl Babies

By Martin Waddell

## Curriculum links

- SEAL – new beginnings / relationships

- Narrative unit – stories with predictive pattern

- Geography – habitats

- Science – nocturnal animals

- Maths – counting

- Topics – animals / into the woods / mini-beasts / all about me

## *Session 1*

## Introduction

*Sit around the story square.*

Recap on group rules:

Go through story components (who, where, when, what happened, the end) linked to general everyday things (who did you walk to school with? etc.)

Introduce the book 'Owl Babies' and flick through the pages with a brief summary . . . do not go to the end.

Describe how session will run and content of session.

Developing:
- Understanding group rules
- Understanding story components
- Familiarity of story

## Warm up

*Stuck-in-the-mud-style game . . .*

Two children are the owls and the other children are mini-beasts / small insects. The children run around the room . . . the owls have to tag the mini-beasts. If tagged, the child has to stand still with arms out. The child can be freed/rescued by another child crawling through his or her legs.

Emphasise the words 'predator' (owl) and 'prey' (mini-beasts/insects).

Developing:
- Attention
- Specific topic vocabulary
- Group cohesion

## Focus one

### *Story and predictions*

Read most of the story but not all. . . . Ask the children, 'Where do you think their mummy went?'

The children are to then get into small groups and decide where the mummy has gone and act it out (maybe collecting worms, finding twigs, etc.).

The children then show other groups their role-play and idea around where mummy went.

Developing:
- Story familiarity
- Prediction and inference skills
- Social skills; group cohesion/group skills
- Feedback to others
- Expressive and receptive language
- 'Where' component

Other groups are asked to comment on something about the role-play of the group they watched that they liked/enjoyed.

## Focus two

### *Hoop nests*

Get some hoops (if there are no hoops, then use string/rope/wool and make circles on the floor). Spread them around the room.

Children are told these hoops are 'nests' that the children now have to fly around the room – generate synonyms for 'fly' together as a group: swoop/glide/sail/soar/flap.

Developing:
- Attention and listening
- Vocabulary extension
- Number language/ counting
- Social skills
- Rehearsal of specific line from story

The practitioner narrates as the children fly: 'Look at Ted soaring through the air,' etc. When the practitioner shouts 'nest,' the children have to find a nest and jump into it.

Ask a child to say a word to describe what he or she was doing – encouraging a synonym for 'fly.'

When children are in a nest, get them all to shout out at the same time the line repeated in story: 'I want my mummy!'

Extension: change the number of children (owls) to go into the nest so when the practitioner starts again, they say, 'This time I am *adding* an owl baby. . . . I need two owl babies in the nest when you stop.'

## Completion

### Sit around story square.

Recap and review:

> Go through the story components: who, where, when, what happened.
>
> Discuss the ending (which they haven't got to yet).
>
> What do they think will happen?

Developing:
- Story component understanding
- Prediction and expression skills

Everyone have a pretend shower: wash off the session and de-roll.

## Session 2

### Introduction

### Sit around the story square.

Recap on group rules:

> Go through story components: who, where, when, what happened.
>
> Describe how session will run and content of session.

Developing:
- Understanding group rules
- Understanding story components

## Warm up

Choose a warm-up activity from those listed in the warm-up section.

## Focus one

### *Different endings*

Remind the children that they don't know the ending to the story yet. The children are to give three different ideas on how the story might end.

Developing:

- Prediction skills
- Expressive language skills
- Social skills; conversation skills/ turn taking/ negotiation
- 'The end' component

The children are put into groups and then act out together with some dialogue, if possible, an ending scene. Show the other groups.

## Focus two

### *Story square*

Acting out the book of 'Owl Babies' . . .

This story has speaking parts, so children can copy the lines from the book as they are read and prompted through the practitioner.

Developing:

- Attention and Listening
- Story understanding
- Narrative development
- Processing
- Sequencing
- Spoken language recall
- Social Skills: eye contact/ sharing space & cooperation/NVC

Make the story square more of a circle in this activity, and tell the children they are the nest surrounding the baby owls.

## Completion

### *Sit around story square.*

Recap and review:

Go through the story components:

Who, where, when, what happened, the end.

Developing

- Story component understanding
- Story understanding

Everyone have a pretend shower: wash off the session and de-roll.

## The Frog Prince

By Brothers Grimm

### Curriculum links

- SEAL – relationships / changes / getting on and falling out

- Narrative unit – traditional and fairy tales / stories by the same author

- Science – amphibians / life cycles

- Topics – animals / pond life / once upon a time

## *Session 1*

## Introduction

### *Sit around the story square.*

Go through story components about general things with children (who, where, when, what happened, the end).

Recap on group rules:

> Introduce 'The Frog Prince' story and describe how session will run and content of session.

Read story.

Developing:
- Understanding group rules
- Understanding story components
- Familiarity of story

## Warm Up

### *Name catch*

From warm-up section, say, 'Ball is a golden ball!'

## Focus one

### *Moral of the story*

Discuss . . .

'What you have promised, you must do.'

Discuss: What is a promise?

Was Princess right to make a promise she never meant to keep?

Was her father right to make her keep the promise even though she didn't mean it?

What could Princess have done as a different way of making things right with the frog if she really felt she couldn't fulfil her promise?

What promise have the children made before?

**Developing:**

- Developing understanding of story
- Social skills: pair work/ ee contact/ turn taking
- Feelings vocabulary extension
- Higher level language and verbal reasoning

Get into pairs – the children are to freeze-frame three scenes together. All the children are given the scene and then given one minute to work together to make it into a freeze frame – the practitioner then tells everybody, 'Time up in three, two, one . . . freeze frame.'

Scenes they can do:

Princess promising to take the frog home by the pond / Princess running away with ball and without frog / King answering the door to the frog / King telling Princess she must keep her promise / Princess sharing her food with the frog / Princess taking the frog to bed / The frog transforming into a prince.

Practitioner commentates on the presentation of the children's freeze frame: 'Amber is the princess, and she looks upset, sad; can anyone think of more words?'

'Maddy is the king . . . her face looks angry. . . .'

## Focus two

### Transformations

Discuss the word 'transform' – encourage children to generate similar words to this: change, evolve, etc.

Ask children to think of other stories with transformations:

Ugly duckling into a swan

Cinderella, servant into a princess

Regular turtles into Teenage Mutant Ninja Turtles

Snow White's wicked queen into an old lady

Transformers from robots into cars . . .

Developing:
- Attention
- Story links
- Verb Vocabulary
- Sentence completion
- Memory

The children all find a space and curl up into a ball on the floor, and they decide what they are going to transform into. Then slowly they uncurl and transform into something and make the shape.

The practitioner can go around and tap children on the shoulder. They should form the sentence 'I have transformed into a . . .' (the children can say 'changed' if 'transformed' is too difficult).

Once they say what they have transformed into, ask them to say two things that the item/person/animal can do – e.g. truck ('drive and beep horn'), giraffe ('eat and walk') etc.

Extension: the children come together at the end of the activity and sit around the story square. Can they remember what their peers turned into? 'Melody, can you tell me what Eleanor transformed into?'

## Completion

*Sit around story square.*

Recap and review:

>   Go through the story components: who, where, when, what happened, the end.

Everyone shake off session and de-roll.

Developing:
- Story component understanding
- Expressive language skills

## Session 2

### Introduction

*Sit around the story square.*

Go through story components about 'The Frog Prince' (who, where, when, what happened, the end).

Recap on group rules:

Recap on what a promise is.

> Developing:
> - Understanding group rules
> - Understanding story components
> - Familiarity of story

### Warm up

*Vocabulary ball roll*

From warm-up section, say, 'Ball is a golden ball!'

### Focus one

*Dinner scene*

Three children at the table:

As characters: King, the frog and Princess.

Other children pretend to be waiters – they come up to the table one by one and offer a plate of food (the child playing a waiter makes up what is on the plate).

They are encouraged to pretend to carry a tray, and the practitioner asks if the tray is heavy or light (if it is light, they carry it above their head; if it is heavy, they carry it low down).

> Developing:
> - Attention
> - Food vocabulary
> - Heavy/light concepts
> - Social interactions: entering an interaction/ eye contact
> - Use of 'because'

The character being offered food has to decide if he or she wants to eat it or not and respond in a sentence. If he or she says yes or no, the practitioner then encourages an explanation starting with 'because.'

For example:

*Waiter:* 'Would you like this spaghetti bolognaise?'
*King:* 'No thank you.'

Asked why:

*King:* 'Because I don't like pasta.'

## Focus two

### Story square

Acting out 'The Frog Prince' . . .

This story has speaking parts so children can copy the lines from the book as they are read.

## Completion

### Sit around story square.

Recap and review:

Go through the story components: who, where, when, what happened, the end.

Say their favourite part of the story.

Developing:

- Attention and Listening
- Story understanding
- Narrative development
- Processing
- Sequencing
- Spoken language recall
- Social Skills: eye contact/ sharing space & cooperation/ NVC

Developing:

- Story component understanding
- Expressive language

Everyone have a pretend shower: wash off the session and de-roll.

## The Three Billy Goats Gruff

By Paul Galdone

### Curriculum links

- SEAL – no to bullying

- Narrative unit – traditional and fairy tales / predictive and patterned language

- Science – bridge building / materials / growing grass

- Maths – size order

- Topics – animals / on the farm / once upon a time

## Session 1

### Introduction

*Sit around the story square.*

Go through the story components about general things with children (who, where, when, what happened, the end).

Recap on group rules:

Introduce 'The Three Billy Goats' story and describe how session will run and content of session.

Read story.

Developing:

- Understanding group rules
- Understanding story components
- Familiarity of story

### Warm up

*In the river / on the bank*

A piece of string is laid out on the floor. The children stand on one side.

Explain to the children that one side of the string is 'the river' and the other side is 'the bank.' All the children start by lining up behind the string.

Developing:

- Attention and Listening
- 'Where' component

Tell them they are standing on the side of 'the bank.' When you call the word 'river,' they must all jump to the other side. When you call 'bank,' they jump back. The children are out when they end up on the side of 'the river' when they should be on 'the bank' or vice versa. To make things more difficult, speed up the commands, having the children go faster and faster with each call. You can also give them a series of commands such as 'river, river, bank, river,' so they would jump twice for each river, then once over to 'bank' and back again . . .

Ask the children at the end, 'where' were they jumping?

## Focus one and two

### *Hot Seating – teacher in role*

The practitioner is the Troll (or use a Troll puppet).

The children try to discover why the Troll is so grumpy and mean . . .

The children are to ask questions: 'Why are you sad/grumpy/mean?'

Encourage children to think of a solution to tell the Troll.

Activities can be carried out to follow on from the scenarios the Troll has created:

Developing:

- Asking questions
- Reasoning skills
- Problem solving
- Vocabulary
- Social interactions/ making friends/ eye contact/ Social skills

'It's horrible living under a bridge': children can create a new house – split into groups and physically make a house together: walls / door / window / flowers / swimming pool. Once the children have made house, they tell everyone what part of the house they are.

'I have a headache because the goats are so noisy.'

Children re-create a bridge with children opposite each other in two lines.

Each person has to go over the bridge as quietly as possible with the Troll sending them back if they are too noisy.

(Emphasise noisy and quiet vocabulary.)

'I have no friends.'

Everyone can decide to throw a party for the Troll and generate vocabulary around what can be at the party.

Each child then approaches the Troll and tries to make friends with the Troll – introduce self, ask him a question, invite him to something, say something nice and so on. The practitioner can go through different things the children could say and facilitate if they find this difficult.

## Completion

*Sit around story square.*

Recap and review:

> Go through the story components: who, where, when, what happened, the end.

> Say their favourite part of the focus activities.

Developing:
- Story component understanding
- Expressive language

Everyone have a pretend shower: wash off the session and de-roll.

## Session 2

### Introduction

*Sit around the story square.*

Go through story components about 'The Three Billy Goats Gruff' story (who, where, when, what happened, the end).

Recap on group rules:

Recap/discuss the reasons that the Troll behaved the way he did – thinking about last session and scenarios that were produced.

Developing:
- Understanding group rules
- Understanding story components
- Familiarity of story

### Warm up

Choose a warm-up activity from the warm-up section.

### Focus one

*Character game*

Children name 'who' in story and create a position for that character – for example:

Troll – pretending to crouch under bridge

Little billy goat – squeeze into small ball

Medium billy goat – on all fours

Big billy goat – make self-big and charge!

Children walk round the room, and the practitioner shouts 'stop,' then says the name of a character, and the children get into that position – the last child to get into position is out (that child can then take the practitioner role for the next round).

Extend: add a phrase to each character.

Developing:
- Attention and listening
- 'Who' component
- Expressive sentence rehearsal

## Focus two

### Story bridge

Acting out 'The Three Billy Goats Gruff' story . . .

Make a bridge rather than the story square . . .

Make two sides of a bridge – children sit opposite each other instead of a square for this story

This story has speaking parts, so children can copy the lines from the book as they are read.

Developing:
- Attention and Listening
- Story understanding
- Narrative development
- Processing
- Sequencing
- Spoken language recall
- Social Skills: eye contact/ sharing space & cooperation/ NVC

## Completion

### Sit around story square.

Recap and review:

Go through the story components: who, where, when, what happened, the end.

Recap which child went over first and then next and then last. Facilitator should emphasise these concepts.

Everyone have a pretend shower: wash off the session and de-roll.

> Developing:
> - Story component understanding
> - Expressive language
> - First-Next-Last recap

## Additional activities or alternatives

### First – next – last

The children are put into groups of three. They decide between themselves who will go first, next and last over the bridge.

Recreate a bridge (again children make two lines facing each other with a pretend bridge in the middle).

They then walk along the bridge one after the other – extend by asking them to all walk down the bridge in various ways: like a Troll, like a goat, happy, sad, angry, hungry, etc.

> Developing:
> - Expressive/ negotiation skills
> - Social skills
> - Sequencing
> - Vocabulary understanding
> - First/middle/last concept understanding and use

The other children must then label who went first, middle or last:

'Ellis was first . . . Luke was next and Emily was last.'

## Cleversticks

By Bernard Ashley

### Curriculum links

- SEAL – good to be me / new beginnings / living in the wider world

- Narrative unit – stories from different cultures

- Geography – different cultures and eating/foods

- Topics – marvellous me / starting school / exploring different traditions

## *Session 1*

### Introduction

*Sit around the story square.*

Recap on group rules:

Go through story components about starting school with children – e.g.:

Who was their first teacher?

Who did they walk to school with?

Where was their classroom?

When did they start school?

What happened on their first day?

What did they tell their mums/dads at the end of their first day?

Extend: How did they feel?

Developing:
- Understanding group rules
- Understanding story components
- Familiarity of story
- Sentence formulation

Introduce 'Cleversticks' story (about being good at some things and needing help with others) and describe how session will run and content of session.

### Warm up

#### *Alliteration Names*

From warm-up section to support 'good to be me' theme.

### Focus one

#### *Story square*

Acting out 'Cleversticks' . . .

This story has speaking parts so children can copy the lines from the book as they are read.

Developing:
- Attention and Listening
- Story understanding
- Narrative development
- Processing
- Sequencing
- Spoken language recall
- Social Skills: eye contact/ sharing space & cooperation/ NVC

## Focus two

### *'I can'*

The children get into a circle. One child goes into the centre, acts out something he or she can do or is good at, and then says, e.g., a sentence: 'I am good at horse riding.'

Everyone claps and says 'well done' together.

Then another child goes into the middle, and this repeats until everyone has a turn.

Extend: go around again with each child going into the circle. This time they go into the circle and choose one of the things that have been said that they aren't as good at.

Developing:

- Attention and listening
- Social skills/ cohesion/ taking turns
- Social language rehearsal
- Memory

The child who can do that joins them in the circle and says, 'I can help – copy me,' and then the children act out that skill together . . . everyone claps.

## Completion

### *Sit around story square.*

Recap and review:

Story components from 'Cleversticks.'

Go through:

Developing:

- Story component understanding
- Expressive language
- Sequencing

who, where, when, what happened, the end.

Everyone shake off session and de-roll.

## Additional activities or alternatives

### *Eating differently*

Discuss together different ways to eat food:

Knife and fork

Spoon

Chopsticks

Hands

Bread / chapatti.

> Developing:
> - Vocabulary
> - Attention

Everyone sits around a pretend table, when the practitioner shouts

out one of the ways to eat . . . and everyone pretends to eat this way.

The practitioner randomly asks children what they are eating

## The Gingerbread Man

### Curriculum links

- SEAL – going for goals

- Narrative unit – predictable and patterned language / traditional tale

- Food technology / science – cooking gingerbread

- Science – sinking and floating

- Topics – fables / animals / on the farm / once upon a time . . .

## Session 1

Introduction

*Sit around the story square.*

Recap on group rules:

Introduce story 'The Gingerbread Man' –
show some of the pictures . . . ask the
children to predict story components (who,
where, when, what happened, the end) from
pictures or past knowledge of the story.

> Developing:
> - Understanding group rules
> - Understanding story components
> - Familiarity of story

Note – the name of the author of this story is unknown . . .

Discuss the Gingerbread Man 'bragging' – what was the Gingerbread Man trying to do?

Describe how session will run and content of session.

## Warm up

### Can I cross your river, Mr Fox?

One child is elected to be the 'Fox' and stands with his or her back turned. The rest of the children stand about 5 metres away in a line facing the back of 'Fox.' Altogether the children chant, 'Fox, Fox, may we cross your shining river?' The

Developing:
- Attention and Listening
- Vocabulary
- Sentence rehearsal

'Fox' answers, 'Not unless you wear the colour red,' or, 'Not unless you are wearing black shoes.' If the children are wearing those items, they have to run across to the side where 'Fox' is before 'Fox' turns around and catches them. Any child that is caught running across can either be the new 'Fox' or has to go back to the start and try again.

## Focus one

### What if?

Ask the children questions, such as: what other choices could the Gingerbread Man have made other than climbing on the fox's back?

Developing:
- Verbal reasoning
- Prediction and inference
- Social skills/ group skills
- Expressive language
- 'The end' component
- 'What' component

The children are to get into groups and act out a different choice that the Gingerbread Man made and therefore what happened next . . . and change the end.

Show other groups at the end.

## Focus two

### Story square

Acting out 'The Gingerbread Man' . . .

This story has speaking parts, so children can copy the lines from the book as they are read.

Encourage all the children in and around the square to copy the Gingerbread Man's repetitive line: 'Run, run as fast as you can! You can't catch me. I'm the Gingerbread Man!'

## Completion

*Sit around story square.*

Recap and review:

> Story components from 'The Gingerbread Man.'

Go through:

> who, where, when, what happened, the end.

Everyone shake off session and de-roll.

Developing:
- Attention and Listening
- Story understanding
- Narrative development
- Processing
- Sequencing
- Spoken language recall
- Social Skills: eye contact/ sharing space & cooperation/ NVC

Developing:
- Story component understanding
- Sequencing
- Expressive language

## Session 2

### Introduction

*Sit around the story square.*

Recap on group rules:

Recap the story 'The Gingerbread Man' (who, where, when, what happened, the end).

Describe how session will run and content of session.

Developing:
- Understanding group rules
- Understanding story components
- Familiarity of story

### Warm up

Select a warm-up activity from the warm-up section.

## Focus one

### *Making a Gingerbread Man*

Pretend to make a Gingerbread Man. . . . The children stand in a circle to make a pretend 'giant bowl.'

Like the story square technique, the practitioner should point at the children to go into the middle (bowl).

Developing:

- Vocabulary (cookery/verb related)
- Attention
- Comprehension
- Sequencing

- 'First shake in the flour' – the children around the circle pretend to shake in flour – one or two children go in the middle

- 'Then throw in some ginger' – one or two children go in the middle, and children in the circle pretend to shake in ginger

- 'Then add a sprinkle of cinnamon'

- 'Add two heaped spoons of baking soda'

- 'A sprinkle of nutmeg'

- 'A pinch of salt'

Be sure children listen to the verb and act it out (shake / sprinkle / pinch / heaped spoons).

- 'Everybody mix these together' – the children around the circle pretend to mix – the children inside the circle move around like they are being mixed!

- 'Turn on the oven' – the circle children pretend to turn a dial

- 'Roll out the dough until it is flat' – the children around the circle pretend to roll – the children inside the circle roll around and then are encourage to lie flat once they think they have been rolled enough!

- 'Bake for ten minutes . . . everybody count to 10.'

- 'And now we have Gingerbread Men' – the children find a space and make a Gingerbread Man pose.

## Focus two

### *Float or sink?*

Discuss how things float and sink – link to words 'heavy' and 'light.'

Discuss materials more likely to sink (metal) and float (wood).

Developing:

- Attention and Listening
- Vocabulary/concepts around sink and float
- Processing
- Prediction

The children are to walk around the room, and, when practitioner shouts 'freeze,' the children stop. The practitioner shouts out an item . . . if the children think it will float, they stick their arms out and pretend to float . . . if they think it will sink, they sink down to the floor.

Examples of items:

Stone / brick / book / Gingerbread Man / television / chair / car / iron / keys / leaf / crisp packet / feather / ice / boat / armband / rubber duck / sponge.

## Completion

### *Sit around story square.*

Recap and review:

Story components from Gingerbread Man.

Go through:

who, where, when, what happened, the end.

Developing:

- Story component understanding
- Sequencing
- Story review
- Expressive language

Everyone shake off session and de-roll.

## Funnybones

By Janet and Allen Ahlberg

### Curriculum links

- SEAL – good to be me / health and well-being

- Narrative unit – fantasy

- Science – bones / human body
- Topics – all about me / Halloween / animals

## Session 1

## Introduction

*Sit around the story square.*

Recap on group rules:

Introduce story 'Funnybones' – show some pictures . . . ask children to predict story components (who, where, when, what happened, the end) from pictures or past knowledge of the story.

Developing:

- Understanding group rules
- Understanding story components
- Familiarity of story
- Prediction and Inference

Describe how session will run and content of session.

## Warm up

*Body to body*

The children walk around room. The practitioner shouts 'stop' and will say a part of the body to match with someone else's:

'foot to foot'

'arm to arm'

'head to head'

'hand to hand'

'finger to finger'

'back to back'

and so on . . .

Developing:

- Attention and Listening
- Body part vocabulary
- Social skills; cohesion/ eye contact
- Processing

Children have to find someone as quickly as possible to match their body part to. If it is an uneven number, then the person needs to find a pair to join and put three body parts together.

The practitioner can ask a different child each time to shout out the body part to body part.

The practitioner can also speed up instructions and give children more body parts whilst still in their pair: 'toe to toe . . . now hand to hand . . . now bottom to bottom!'

## Focus one

### *Story square*

Acting out 'Funnybones' . . .

This story has speaking parts so children can copy the lines from the book as they are read.

The beginning of the story is setting the scene. Start with all the children on one side of the room, and practitioner narrates the story . . . the children walk and follow the practitioner and go on a journey.

They move slowly towards the story square . . . moving slowly, walking along a 'dark dark hill' (exaggerate as if climbing a hill) . . . then town . . . street . . . house (open door) . . . down staircase (walk as if going down stairs and into a cellar – all sit around the story square).

Developing:

- Attention and Listening
- Story understanding
- Narrative development
- Processing
- Sequencing
- Spoken language recall
- Social Skills: eye contact/ sharing space & cooperation/ NVC

From this point, start acting out in the story square as skeletons are introduced.

## Focus two

### *Frightening fun*

Discuss with the children the different ways the skeletons tried to frighten each other. First think of a different word for 'frightened' (scared/terrified/fear/petrify/shock).

In threes, children take the roles of the two skeletons and the dog and try different ways of scaring each other. Ask them if they can act as though they are not expecting to be surprised.

**Developing:**
- Vocabulary
- Social skills; cohesion/ turn taking/ eye contact
- Expressive language

Ask the children at the end to say how they frightened someone, e.g. 'I jumped out from behind a tree' or 'I pulled a funny face.'

## Completion

*Sit around story square.*

Recap and review:

Story components from 'Funnybones' . . .

Go through:

who, where, when, what happened, the end.

**Developing:**
- Story component understanding
- Sequencing
- Story review
- Expressive language

Everyone sing a song together:

'The foot bone's connected to the leg bone . . . the leg bone's connected to the hip bone' . . . etc. (Ideally use the song 'Dem Bones' by James Weldon Johnson.)

Everyone shake off session and de-roll.

## Session 2

### Introduction

*Sit around the story square.*

Recap on group rules:

**Developing:**
- Understanding group rules
- Understanding story components
- Familiarity of story

Story components around 'Funnybones' (who, where, when, what happened, the end).

Describe how session will run and content of session.

## Warm up

### Lead with your . . .

The children are asked to walk around the room but to lead their bodies with certain parts of their body. Discuss the meaning of the word 'lead.'

The practitioner shouts this instruction: 'Leading with your head' (children will therefore stick their heads out further and walk around like this). The practitioner changes instruction: 'Leading with your arm/bottom/ear/etc.'

Developing:

- Attention and Listening
- Body vocabulary
- Processing

Can increase speed of changing body parts.

## Focus one

### Skeleton scenes

Recap the story with the children and pick out a selection of scenes – i.e. the skeletons playing in that park, taking a ride on the Ghost Train.

Split the children up into small groups and ask them to choose their favourite scene, and then ask them to create a still image.

Once the children have practiced their still image, the practitioner turns this activity into a game of musical statues, where the group to organise their still scene the fastest is the winner.

Developing:

- Attention and Listening
- Story review
- Social skills; cohesion/ turn taking/ negotiation
- Expressive language
- 'What happened' component

## Focus two

### Bone names

Four corners of the room are to be labelled with different bone names (with pictures to support) – go through the real names of the bones with the children:

Head – skull

Back – spine

Upper arm – humerus

Upper leg – femur.

> Developing:
> - Attention and Listening
> - Bone vocabulary

The children dance to some music (ideally the song 'Dem Bones') – when the music stops, they run over to a corner in the room. With the practitioner's back turned, they call a name of a corner – anyone standing in that corner is out, and the game carries on until you are down to three children (at this point you can eliminate a corner, same again when down to two).

You keep playing until you have one outright winner. Alternatively, to avoid eliminating anyone, you can reward points to the children who are standing in the chosen corner. The child with the most points at the end of the game is the winner.

## Completion

### Sit around story square.

Recap and review:

> Developing:
> - Story component understanding
> - Sequencing
> - Story review
> - Expressive language

Story components from 'Funnybones.'
Go through:

who, where, when, what happened,
the end.

Everyone sing a song together: 'The foot bone's connected to the leg bone . . . the leg bone's connected to the hip bone.'

Everyone shake off session and de-roll.

## Whatever Next

By Jill Murphy

**Curriculum links**

- SEAL – going for goals

- Narrative unit – stories with familiar settings / stories by the same author

- Science – space

- Topics – bears, explorers, space, transport

## *Session 1*

## Introduction

*Sit around the story square.*

Recap on group rules:

Introduce story and show front cover.

Story components around what children think might happen in story just from this (who, where, when, what happened, the end).

Describe how session will run and content of session.

Developing:

- Understanding group rules
- Understanding story components
- Familiarity of story
- Prediction
- Expressive language

## Warm up

Choose a warm-up game from warm-up section.

## Focus one

## *Transport group*

Split children into small groups. The practitioner can use real boxes or pretend boxes . . .

Developing:

- Transport vocabulary
- Sequencing
- Expressive language
- Social skills; negotiation/ cohesion/ turn taking

The members of the group have to decide what transport their box is going to turn into (in the story, the box is turned into a rocket). Then act it out all together (e.g. car / ride at the fair / airplane / train). The children should be encouraged to think about how they get in / what they do when in / how the transport moves – all together.

They should then decide where their transport is going and what they will do when they are there.

Encourage conversation skills with each other and language around transport. Get them to think and describe the sequence of how we get into and use transport.

Show the other groups once complete.

## Focus two

### Story square

Acting out 'Whatever Next' . . .

This story has speaking parts so children can copy the lines from the book as they are read.

## Completion

### Sit around story square.

Recap and review:

Story components from 'Whatever Next.' Go through:

who, where, when, what happened, the end.

Developing:

- Attention and Listening
- Story understanding
- Narrative development
- Processing
- Sequencing
- Spoken language recall
- Social Skills: eye contact/ sharing space & cooperation/ NVC

Developing:

- Story component understanding
- Sequencing
- Story review
- Expressive language

Everyone shower off session and de-roll.

## Session 2

### Introduction

### Sit around the story square.

Recap on group rules:

Recap story components around 'Whatever Next' (who, where, when, what happened, the end).

Developing:

- Understanding group rules
- Understanding story components
- Familiarity of story
- Expressive language

Describe how session will run and content of session.

## Warm up

Choose a warm-up game from the warm-up section.

## Focus one

### Trip to the moon

The practitioner facilitates packing a rocket ready for everyone to take off to the moon.

The children are encouraged to pack what they think will be useful.

Once everyone has said something, the practitioner tells the children that they can fit only five things into the rocket . . . what are the five most important things?

Developing:

- Vocabulary
- Expressive language/ use of because
- Verbal reasoning
- Negotiation

Encourage children to name an item and to give a reason. Ask other children to raise their hands if they agree . . . eventually pack five items that the group members have decided on together (with facilitation).

End of activity: everyone climb into the rocket and count down: '5, 4, 3, 2, 1, blast off,' and jump up into the air.

## Focus two

### Moonwalking

The children are to walk around the room like they are on the moon (slowly and exaggerated). The

Developing:

- Attention and Listening
- Comprehension
- Position/ direction concepts
- Vocabulary (planets/space)

practitioner shouts out instructions for all children to follow but to carry out in 'moonwalking' mode (slow motion).

Instructions should contain direction language:

'Everyone move forwards . . . go left . . . walk backwards . . . go right . . . walk next to someone else . . .'

Extension: to start the activity, everybody 'gets into the rocket' and blasts off into space – as the children travel through space, they name planets or things related to space that they see – the practitioner facilitates this.

## Completion

*Sit around story square.*

Recap and review:

> Discuss how little bear wanted to go to the moon and so used his imagination to get there . . . where would the children really like to go?

Developing:
- Story component understanding
- 'Where' component
- Story review
- Expressive language

Everyone shake off session and de-roll.

## Handa's Surprise
By Eileen Browne

**Curriculum links**

- SEAL/PHSE – relationships / healthy eating

- Narrative unit – stories from different cultures

- Maths – heavy/light and subtraction

- Topics – Africa / around the world / explorers / animals / marvellous me

## Session 1

### Introduction

*Sit around the story square.*

Recap on group rules:

Introduce story and show front cover and read first two pages . . .

Story components around what children think might happen in story just from this (who, where, when, what happened, the end).

Describe how session will run and content of session.

Developing:

- Understanding group rules
- Understanding story components
- Familiarity of story
- Prediction
- Expressive language

### Warm up

*Fruit salad!*

Place chairs around the story square: one chair fewer than the total number of players.

Nominate a player to be 'in,' and that player stands in the middle.

Developing:

- Attention and Listening
- Fruit vocabulary

Divide all players into three groups of fruit by going around the circle and naming them: mango, pineapple or banana.

The player who is 'in' calls the name of a fruit. If the player calls out 'mangos,' everyone who is that fruit must get up quickly and change places. Players who are not mangos remain seated.

The person who is 'in' tries to sit in an empty spot whenever players swap positions.

If the player manages to sit in a chair, the player not sitting in a chair is then 'in.' The person in the middle can also call 'fruit salad,' and everyone who is seated has to change spots.

Stop halfway through, and change the fruit to the other fruits that appear in the book.

## Focus one

### Character game

The children name the animals in the book (zebra, ostrich, elephant, monkey, giraffe, antelope, goat, parrot).

Every animal is to be described on how they look and move (giraffe: tall / long neck / big eyes / fast / thin). Encourage the use of describing vocabulary.

Developing:
- Attention and Listening
- Animal vocabulary
- Describing vocabulary
- 'Who' component

The children are to walk around the room as that animal when the practitioner shouts it out. The practitioner reinforces and models vocabulary – e.g. everyone is pretending to be elephant, and the practitioner commentates: 'Everyone is walking around with their long trunks and their big stomping feet. Everyone looks very big and everyone is moving slowly.'

As the children walk around, show them the page of the animal they are acting out and tell them the fruit the animal takes.

## Focus two

### Gifts

The children sit around the story square. The practitioner discusses how the story is about giving a gift to Handa's friend . . . ask the following questions:

Has anyone given someone a present before?

How does it feel when you give someone a present?

Developing:
- Attention
- Vocabulary description skills
- Comprehension
- Expressive language
- Social skills; taking turns
- Memory

Why do you give someone a present?

Start an activity where a child sitting around the square passes a pretend gift to the child next to him or her. That child pretends to open up the box (commentate and encourage the child to be imaginative opening the box – untie ribbon, rip it open fast, slow, peek inside etc.).

As the child looks inside the box, the child that has given the gift describes it without saying its name . . . the person opening the gift then guesses what it is.

Extension: at the end . . . go around the children and ask them if they can remember what gift other children received.

## Completion

*Sit around story square.*

Recap and review:

> Discuss favourite part of the session. Review the animals in the story and what fruit each animal took – can the children remember?

Developing:
- Story review
- Expressive language
- Memory

Everyone shake off session and de-roll.

## *Session 2*

### Introduction

*Sit around the story square.*

Recap on group rules:

Review story and last session.

Describe how session will run and content of session.

Developing:
- Understanding group rules
- Familiarity of story
- Expressive language

## Warm up

### Heavy/light

Discuss the basket from the story and why the basket becomes lighter . . .

The children walk around the room pretending to carry fruit on their heads. When the practitioner says 'heavy,' the children walk like the basket is heavy (encourage them to describe how this will look physically and the facial expressions).

Developing:

- Attention and Listening
- Food vocabulary
- Describing skills
- Heavy/light concept
- Differentiation/Categorisation
- Processing

When the practitioner shouts out 'light,' the children walk like the basket is light.

As the children are walking around, the practitioner also shouts out different foods. If they are healthy foods, then the children continue to walk around.

If the practitioner shouts out a food that is unhealthy, the children sit down as quick as they can.

## Focus one

### Dressing

Discuss where the story is and that the weather is hot . . . think of synonyms for hot (boiling/sweltering/burning/roasting . . .).

Developing:

- Vocabulary: weather and clothes
- Hot and Cold concepts
- 'Where' component

Children to generate clothes that you wear when it's hot.

The children then stand up and pretend to get dressed into clothes that are for hot weather. Children randomly chosen are to tell everyone what items they are wearing.

Go for a walk following each other in a line, pretend to be very hot, and shout out words for 'hot.'

Discuss the opposite of 'hot,' and name some places that have cold weather. . . . Think of other words for 'cold' (freezing/chilly/icy . . .). The children are to name clothes you wear when it is cold.

The children then stand up and pretend to get dressed into clothes that are for cold weather. Children are randomly chosen to tell everyone what items they are wearing.

Go for a walk following each other in a line, pretend to be very cold, and shout out words for 'cold.'

Extension: the children can name the countries they are walking around – naming typically hot countries and typically cold countries – emphasising 'where' the children are.

## Focus two

### Question-mark story square

This time read the story around the square but do not get into the middle.

Discuss what questions are and what question marks look like.

Developing:
- Attention and Listening
- Punctuation awareness
- Question awareness
- Story familiarity

Everyone practice making the shape of one with their hands: start at the top, curve the hand round and down, and then punch forward to make the dot.

Encourage children to then do the question mark action every time there is a question in the story.

'Handa's Surprise' has many questions in it.

## Completion

### Sit around story square.

Recap and review:

Story components from 'Handa's Surprise.' Go through: who, where, when, what happened, the end.

Developing:
- Story component understanding
- Sequencing
- Story review
- Expressive language

Everyone shower off session and de-roll.

## The Ugly Duckling

By Hans Christian Anderson

### Curriculum links

- SEAL/PHSE – new beginnings / getting on and falling out / changes / relationships

- Narrative unit – traditional tales / stories by the same author

- Science – transformations / growth and change / seasons

- Topics – marvellous me / animals / on the farm

## *Session 1*

### Introduction

*Sit around the story square.*

Recap on group rules:

Introduce story . . . ask children if they know it.

Use story components to help children predict how the story may unfold (who, where, when, what happened, the end).

Developing:

- Understanding group rules
- Familiarity of story
- Understanding and use of story components
- Prediction

Describe how session will run and content of session.

### Warm up

*Group game*

Explain that in the story 'The Ugly Duckling,' the duckling is left out and doesn't feel like he belongs.

Developing:

- Social skills
- Group Cohesion

Choose a warm-up game from the warm-up section that is about taking turns / everyone joining in to emphasise that this is important and for the children to experience a game where everyone joins in and works together.

## Focus one

### Egg hatch

The children are to get down to the floor and curl up like they are in an egg. They should generate words around how they feel inside the egg: warm, safe, secure, squashed, sleepy, etc.

Developing:
- Attention
- Vocabulary: emotions

Children then act out 'hatching' from the egg . . . they should generate words once they have hatched to describe how they might feel now: cold, unsure, confused, hungry, excited, happy, scared. . . .

## Focus two

### Story square

Acting out 'The Ugly Duckling' . . .

This story has speaking parts so children can copy the lines from the book as they are read.

Developing:
- Attention and listening
- Story Understanding
- Narrative development
- Processing
- Spoken language recall
- Vocabulary: seasons/weather
- Social Skills
- 'When' component: seasons

Emphasise the change of seasons in the story and get children sitting around the square to make sounds and act out the weather of the seasons. (The practitioner may need to go through the meaning of seasons and the characteristics of seasons in order to familiarise children before they start the story in the story square.)

For example: start in the summer with egg hatching – sun shining. . . . Move on to autumn and duckling being left out by others, and then winter ducks fly away, spring arrives, and duckling has transformed.

## Completion

*Sit around story square.*

Recap and review:

> Story components from 'The Ugly Duckling.'

> Go through: who, where, when, what happened, the end.

Developing:
- Story component understanding
- Sequencing
- Story review
- Expressive language

Everyone shower off session and de-roll.

## Session 2

### Introduction

*Sit around the story square.*

Recap on group rules:

Recap story. . . . Use story components to help children scaffold story (who, where, when, what happened, the end).

Describe how session will run and content of session.

Developing:
- Understanding group rules
- Familiarity of story
- Understanding and use of story components

### Warm up

*Duckling actions*

The children are to name actions a duckling presents with and then act this out (waddle / fly / paddle / quack / peck).

The practitioner chooses four actions, and then children move around the room. The practitioner then shouts out an action, and

Developing:
- Attention and Listening
- Vocabulary
- Processing

children should move around the room acting out the action and pretending to be a duckling.

The practitioner changes the action throughout the task and can speed up instructions to make the task more challenging.

## Focus one

### *Reflections*

Discuss the word reflection and what it means and where you can see reflections (mirror / glass / window / water). Ask the children, where did the ugly duckling see his reflection?

Developing:

- Attention
- Vocabulary
- Social skills: eye contact/ turn taking/ awareness

The children are to get into pairs, standing opposite each other. One child makes slow movements with his or her hands and slowly extends to moving heads, legs etc. The child's partner stands opposite and copies as if the other child were a reflection. Swap roles so the other partner makes movements first.

## Focus two

### *Joining in*

Discuss how the ugly duckling felt being left out all the time. Generate emotions vocabulary.

Developing:

- Attention and Listening
- Emotions vocabulary
- Social skills: group cohesion/ taking turns/ awareness of others
- Social language and entry to groups and play practice

Move on to discussing how you join in games and how we should let others join in.

The children should think of three times during a game when it is good to ask to join in / let others join in: e.g. at the beginning / at the end of someone's turn / when the activity stops for a short amount of time.

Practice phrases to ask to join in: e.g. 'Can I play?' or 'What are you playing? It looks fun!'

Practice phrases to ask others to join in:

'Do you want to play?'

'You can play after this turn if you want to.'

Split into two groups (more if a large group of children in session).

One group starts playing a game – a good game for this is 'balloon pat' from the warm-up section in this book. This activity is about group cohesion / making sure everyone has a turn.

The practitioner starts the one group off playing this game and explains the rules.

The other group then sits to the side and watches the game. The practitioner then points to a child, and the child should go up to the game and ask to join in. The group allows the child to join, and someone explains the rules to the child quickly.

Evaluate at the end how it feels to join in and to let others join in.

## Completion

*Sit around story square.*

Recap and review:

- Story components from 'The Ugly Duckling': who, where, when, what happened, the end.

- Sing song / play music: 'The Ugly Duckling' by Danny Kaye.

Developing:
- Story component understanding
- Sequencing
- Story review
- Expressive language

Everyone shower off session and de-roll.

# Rosie's Hat

By Julia Donaldson

## Curriculum links

- SEAL/PHSE – changes / relationships / going for goals

- Narrative unit – stories in a familiar setting / stories by the same author

- Topics – marvellous me / beside the seaside / people who help us

## *Session 1*

## Introduction

*Sit around the story square.*

Recap on group rules:

Introduce story . . . ask children if they know it.

Read story to children.

Describe how session will run and content of session.

> Developing:
> - Understanding group rules
> - Familiarity of story

## Warm up

## *Pass the hat*

Use warm-up game 'I can make a sound like this . . .' from the warm-up section. Have a hat: the person making the sound should wear the hat. Then pass the hat onto the next child, and that child makes a sound everyone copies.

## Focus one

## *People-who-help-us character game*

Think of people that help us: fire-fighter, paramedic, police officer, lifeguard, doctor, nurse etc.

Think about what they do, and act out how they present . . . come up with four or five

> Developing:
> - Attention and Listening
> - Vocabulary: people who help us and describing vocabulary

different ones. The children should walk around room. . . . The practitioner then shouts out a character, and children act it out.

Speed up to make it more challenging.

## Focus two

### Story square

Acting out 'Rosie's Hat' . . .

This story has speaking parts, so children can copy the lines from the book as they are read.

Developing:

- Attention and Listening
- Story understanding
- Narrative development
- Processing
- Sequencing
- Spoken language recall
- Social Skills: eye contact/ sharing space & Cooperation/ NVC

## Completion

### Sit around story square.

Recap and review:

> Story components from 'Rosie's Hat': who, where, when, what happened, the end.

Everyone shower off session and de-roll.

Developing:

- Story component understanding
- Sequencing
- Story review
- Expressive language

## Session 2

### Introduction

### Sit around the story square.

Recap on group rules:

Recap story . . . use story components: who, where, when, what happened, the end.

Developing:

- Understanding group rules
- Familiarity of story
- Story components understanding
- Author awareness & links

Discuss Julia Donaldson as an author, and discuss the meaning of the word 'author' – do the children know any other Julia Donaldson books?

Describe how session will run and content of session.

## Warm up

Choose a warm-up game from the warm-up section.

## Focus one

### Photos

Discuss the end of the book 'Rosie's Hat' and that a photo is taken.

The children get into groups and create still images of scenes in the book.

The practitioner comes around and takes a picture with a pretend camera.

Developing:

- Attention
- Memory/recall of scenes
- Social skills: negotiation/ conversation/ turn taking/ cohesion

The children given scenes to do and discuss together how they should create it.

## Focus two

### When I'm older

The children are to think about what they would like to be/do when they are older.

Find a space, and act it out without words.

Give some practice time: this enables the practitioner to help those children who need it.

Developing:

- Attention
- Inference/prediction
- Expressive language
- Vocabulary: jobs/ hobby

The children are to then come and sit around the story square. Every child goes into the middle and acts out what they want to be/do when they are older . . . the other children guess what that job/role is.

Extension: once a child acts out in the square, ask the child to add some words to the performance.

## Completion

*Sit around story square.*

Recap and review the story 'Rosie's Hat.'

Every child comes up with something they enjoyed about the child they are sat next to in terms of their performance from that session.

Developing:
- Story review
- Expressive language
- Social skills – awareness of others/ feedback skills

Everyone shower off session and de-roll.

# Chapter three
# YEAR 2

The following activities are more suited for Year 2 level work and content. However, some Year 1 groups could access these – depending on their language and learning levels. (Equally, Year 2 children can access all the previous sessions in this book, and the following are not exclusive.)

The stories can move on to also having a 'problem' to discuss within the story components. Most stories have a problem to overcome – and this helps extend the children's storytelling.

The stories in this section can also have elements changed to start helping children to create stories and 'innovate' rather than solely 'imitate.'

An example of how a child's own story can then be turned into an entire session is also shown in this section. This is a way children can create their own stories, share them with their peers and see their stories come to life.

## The Owl and the Pussycat
By Edward Lear

### Curriculum links

- SEAL/PHSE – relationships / new beginnings

- Narrative unit – traditional tales / poetry

- Science – weather

- Topics – around the world / explorers / animals / transport

## Session 1

### Introduction

*Sit around the story square.*

Recap on group rules:

Introduce poem . . . ask the children if they know what a poem is.

Think of some words, and see if the children can think of a word that rhymes (cat, log, nine etc.).

Read the poem to the children.

Describe how session will run and content of session.

> Developing:
> - Understanding group rules
> - Familiarity of story
> - Rhyme awareness

### Warm up

*Musical statues*

Play musical statues linking this activity to the owl and the pussycat dancing under the light of the moon.

Extension: ask the children to choose which character they are: the owl or the pussycat. . . . Encourage them to dance like this animal. The practitioner can commentate as they dance and reflect how the children are moving.

> Developing:
> - Attention and listening
> - Story vocabulary

### Focus one

*Words v. non-words*

Pretend everyone is climbing into a boat all together . . . the children put on their life jackets.

Then pretend to sail the sea. . . . The practitioner changes the weather, and the children act how they would be in the boat with that weather.

For example: 'Here comes a fierce storm . . . the waves are crashing . . . everyone hold on!'

Or: 'The sun is shining and the sea is calm . . . everyone is relaxed . . .'

Once the boat gets to the island, everyone climbs ashore and then discusses how in the poem some words have been made up (bong tree / runcible).

Walk around the room (island) listening to words – if the words are real, then keep walking; if a word is made up, then drop to the floor.

Developing:

- Attention and Listening
- Weather vocabulary
- Comprehension
- Real Vs. Non real word awareness

## Focus two

### Five things . . .

Ask the children: 'If you were going away for a year and a day, what five important things would you bring?'

The children list their five things (can be verbal, written down or drawn pictures) and then get into pairs. . . . They compare their lists and complete one list of five items between them, considering each other's items and explaining why they are important.

Developing:

- Social skills; eye contact/ turn taking/ negotiation/ awareness of others.
- Verbal reasoning
- Use of 'because'
- Expressive language

That pair then join another pair and again compare lists and make a joint list . . . continue until the whole group has only one list.

## Completion

### Sit around story square.

Recap and review:

> Story components from 'The Owl and the Pussycat.' Go through:

> who, where, when, what happened, the end.

Developing:

- Story component understanding
- Sequencing
- Story review
- Expressive language

Everyone shower off session and de-roll.

## Session 2

### Introduction

*Sit around the story square.*

Recap on group rules:

Recap what a poem is.

Recap 'The Owl and the Pussycat' . . . who, where, when, what happened, the end.

Developing:

- Understanding group rules
- Familiarity of story
- Rhyme awareness
- Story component understanding
- Sequencing

Describe how session will run and content of session.

## Warm up

### Rhyme clap

Everyone sit around the story square.

Practitioner says a word . . . then shouts out other words . . . if they rhyme with the original word, then the children should clap . . . if it doesn't rhyme, then children don't clap.

Developing:

- Attention and listening
- Phonological awareness – rhyme
- Rhyme generation

Extension: let children take the practitioner roll and come up with different words.

## Focus one

### Role-play

The children are put in pairs:

One child is the pussycat, and the other is the owl.

The practitioner gives the following scenarios to the children:

Developing:

- Attention
- Social skills; eye contact/ conversation/ turn taking.
- Role play skills and NVC
- Negotiation and persuasion language

Pussycat – you don't want to go to sea . . . you don't like water, but you love the owl. What will you eat? Will it be enough money to live on? Where will you go?

Think of three reasons to tell the owl why you shouldn't go.

Owl – persuade the pussycat to come to sea with you. . . . Tell her it's a trip of a lifetime and an adventure. Think of three reasons to tell the cat why you should go.

The children can present to others if they wish at the end of the activity.

## Focus two

### Story square

Acting out 'The Owl and the Pussycat' . . .

This story has speaking parts so children can copy the lines from the book as they are read.

The practitioner can pause at the end of lines to encourage the children sitting around the story square to finish the line in the poem.

Developing:
- Attention and listening
- Story understanding
- Narrative development
- Processing
- Sequencing
- Spoken language recall
- Social skills: eye contact/ sharing space & cooperation/ NVC

## Completion

### Sit around story square.

Recap and review:

> Story components from 'The Owl and the Pussycat.'

> Go through: who, where, when, what happened, the end.

Everyone shake off session and de-roll.

Developing:
- Story component understanding
- Sequencing
- Story review
- Expressive language

## Hairy Maclary

By Lynley Dodd

### Curriculum links

- SEAL/PHSE – getting on and falling out / relationships

- Narrative unit – stories with predictive patterns / poetry

- Science – dog breeds / classification

- Topics – animals / poems

### Session 1

## Introduction

*Sit around the story square.*

Recap on group rules:

Recap what a poem/rhyme is.

The children are to think of a real word or non-real word that rhymes with their names.

Read the story to the children.

Developing:
- Understanding group rules
- Familiarity of story
- Rhyme awareness
- Story component understanding
- Sequencing

## Warm up

*Alliteration names*

See warm-up section for this activity.

## Focus one

*Walk recreation*

Scatter the children around the room, and all together come up with a sentence that rhymes with their names, like in the book – for example:

Jo Palmer who works as a farmer

Amelia Cody who has a friend called Jodi

Isabelle Rox who has lovely locks.

Get one of the children to be the scary character like 'Scarface Claw.'

One child is to start moving around the room and stop as he or she gets to each child, and then that child follows so they create a trail, like in the book, and follow each other collecting the others whilst creating a rhyme – again, similar to the book.

**Developing:**
- Attention and Listening
- Phonological awareness: rhyme
- Sequencing
- Real Vs. Non-word awareness

The practitioner facilitates the rhyme as they walk along . . .

For example: 'Once there was a girl called Jo Palmer who works as a farmer. She went for a walk around her farm to find some friends. . . . First she came across: Amelia Cody who has a friend called Jodi, then around the corner she found Isabelle Rox who has lovely locks . . .' Carry on like this until the 'baddy' jumps out. . . . 'Suddenly Charlie Dickinson the toughest animal on the farm jumped out and chased them all home!'

If there is a name that is very difficult to rhyme, then have staple sentences to use like:

'Jasper Bocas who loved the word Trocas!'

Discuss that this is a non-real word!

## Focus two

### Dog relay

Put the children into small teams, and have a relay race across the room. Each team is given a character (e.g. dog) from the book and have to move like the character during the race (Hercules Morse as big as a horse – big and proud).

**Developing:**
- Attention
- Social skills/ group cohesion
- Describing Vocabulary

The children should generate vocabulary around each of their teams' characters before they race.

## Completion

*Sit around story square.*

Recap and review:

> Story components from 'Hairy Maclary.'

> Go through: who, where, when, what happened, the end.

Everyone shake off session and de-roll.

Developing:
- Story component understanding
- Sequencing
- Story review
- Expressive language

## Dogger

By Shirley Hughes

### Curriculum links

- SEAL/PHSE – Relationships / good to be me

- Narrative unit – stories with familiar settings

- Topics – marvellous me / toys

## Session 1

### Introduction

*Sit around the story square.*

Recap on group rules:

Introduce story and basics of story, including losing something that you love. Ask the children, have they ever lost something they love?

Describe how session will run and content of session.

Developing:
- Understanding group rules
- Familiarity of story

## Warm up

Choose a warm up from the warm-up section.

## Focus one

### Story square

Acting out 'Dogger' . . .

This story has speaking parts, so children can copy the lines from the book as they are read.

Prepare the children to think about what the 'problem' in the story is as the story unfolds . . .

Developing:
- Attention and Listening
- Story understanding
- Narrative development
- Processing
- Sequencing
- Spoken language recall
- Social Skills: eye contact/ sharing space & Cooperation/ NVC

## Focus two

### Summer fair

The children are to find a space in the room and think about a summer fair . . . what activities are there? Each child comes up with an activity (bouncy castle, coconut shy, eating ice cream, tombola, egg and spoon race, raffle, singing etc.).

Developing:
- Attention and listening
- Vocabulary: summer fair vocabulary & describing/ verb vocabulary

The practitioner asks the children what they can do to show this activity (e.g. Practitioner: 'How do we move on a bouncy castle?' Child: 'Jump / fall down').

The children act out the activity all together.

The practitioner models language as children are acting out.

## Completion

*Sit around story square.*

Recap and review:

> Story components from 'Dogger.'
>
> Use story component card: 'Problem' (who, where, when, what happened, problem, the end).

Everyone shake off session and de-roll.

Developing:
- Story component understanding
- Sequencing
- Story review
- Expressive language

## Session 2

### Introduction

*Sit around the story square.*

Recap on group rules:

Recap story 'Dogger' – who, where, when, what happened, problem, the end.

Describe how session will run and content of session.

Developing:
- Understanding group rules
- Familiarity of story
- Story component understanding
- Sequencing

### Warm up

*Ten in the bed*

Children pretend to be in bed like the sister in 'Dogger.'

Lie next to each other in a row and sing, 'Ten in a bed.'

Each time the children sing 'So they all rolled over and one fell out,' one child on the end rolls over and pretends to fall out and then moves away.

Developing:
- Attention
- Subtraction
- Rhyme

## Focus one

### *Blindfold*

One child is blindfolded and stands at one end of the room.

A teddy is placed somewhere in the room. Another child then has to help that child find the teddy.

Developing:
- Attention and listening
- Following and giving instructions
- Direction concepts – understanding and using

The child giving the instructions can give a maximum of only four instructions to get the blindfolded child to the teddy – for example:

Take four steps forward.

Turn to your left.

Take three steps forward.

Take one more step.

Take turns with different children being blindfolded and giving instructions.

## Focus two

### *Story creation*

Sit around the story square and create a story together – similar to 'Dogger' but changing some elements.

Use story components to help plan and sequence: when story starts, main character, what they lose, where they go to look for it, how they find it, the end.

Developing:
- Use of story components
- Sequencing
- Narrative development
- Story recall
- Expressive language
- Story Square Skills

The practitioner notes responses and creates a short story.

Act out the story in the story square.

## Completion

*Sit around story square.*

Recap and review:

Story components from the story the
children have generated and acted
out – go through: who, where, when,
what happened, problem, the end.

Developing:
- Story component understanding
- Sequencing
- Story review
- Expressive language

Everyone shake off session and de-roll.

# The Owl Who Was Afraid of the Dark

By Jill Tomlinson

### Curriculum links

- SEAL – new beginnings / relationships / the wider world

- Narrative unit – stories in familiar setting

- Geography – habitats

- Science – nocturnal animals / light and dark / night and day

- Topics – animals / into the woods / mini-beasts / all about me

## *Session 1*

## Introduction

*Sit around the story square.*

Recap on group rules:

Introduce story and basics of story, including
being afraid of something . . . what are they
scared of?

Developing:
- Understanding group rules
- Familiarity of story

Describe how session will run and content of session.

## Warm up

Choose a warm up from the warm-up section.

## Focus one

### Baby animal names

Discuss how baby owls are called 'owlets.'

What other baby animals have different names?

Generate baby animal names: foal, calf, chick, duckling, puppy, kitten etc.

Developing:

- Attention
- Vocabulary (topic specific)
- Verb vocabulary
- 'Who' component

Ask the children how these animals move and what their actions are (waddle/stride/gallop/creep/bounce/run/jump) and what noises they make . . .

All walk around the room acting out these baby animals.

Split the children into two groups. One group is the audience and watches the other children act out their baby animal of choice, then practitioner asks:

'Who do you think Kitty was acting out?'

The practitioner emphasises 'who.'

## Focus two

### Story square

Acting out 'The Owl Who Was Afraid of the Dark' . . .

This story has speaking parts so children can copy the lines from the book as they are read.

Developing:

- Attention and Listening
- Story understanding
- Narrative development
- Processing
- Spoken language recall
- Social Skills (eye contact/ Communication with others/ sharing space & cooperation/ NVC

## Completion

*Sit around story square.*

Recap and review:

> Story components from 'The Owl Who Was Afraid of the Dark.
>
> Go through: who, where, when, what happened, problem, the end.

Developing:
- Story component understanding
- Sequencing
- Story review
- Expressive language

Everyone shake off session and de-roll.

## Session 2

### Introduction

*Sit around the story square.*

Recap on group rules:

Recap the story 'The Owl Who Was Afraid of the Dark.'

The children are asked to generate words about the dark either from the book or generated themselves . . .

Go around the story square and encourage them to use similar sentences to the ones used in the book:

Dark is . . . beautiful.

Dark is necessary.

Dark is fascinating. . . .

Developing:
- Understanding group rules
- Familiarity of story
- Vocabulary

Describe how session will run and content of session.

### Warm up

Choose a warm up from the warm-up section.

## Focus one

### Nocturnal image of the hour

Discuss the word 'nocturnal' – the practitioner links to the 'when' component and night and day. . . . Discuss animals that are nocturnal like owls (e.g. bat, hedgehog, racoon, koala, tiger, hamster, badger, gerbil etc.).

List some animals that are active in the day.

Developing:
- Vocabulary categorising
- Topic vocabulary
- Processing
- Comprehension
- 'When' component

The children then walk around the room. When the adult shouts 'stop,' all the children stop. The practitioner will say an animal name and the time (morning, afternoon or night), and the children have to act out what that animal would be doing – for example:

'Owl in the afternoon' – children would pretend to sleep sitting in their tree.

'Bat at night' – children would fly around.

'Dog at night' – children would curl up pretending to sleep etc. . . .

## Focus two

### Story creation

Sit around story square and create a story together – similar to 'The Owl Who Was Afraid of the Dark' but changing some elements.

Title of story:

The . . . Who Was Afraid of the . . .

Use story components to help plan and sequence.

The practitioner notes responses and creates a short story.

Act out the story in the story square.

Developing:
- Use of story components
- Sequencing
- Narrative development
- Story recall
- Expressive language
- Story Square skills

## Completion

*Sit around story square.*

Recap and review:

> Story components from the story that the children have generated and acted out.

> Go through: who, where, when, what happened, problem, the end.

Developing:
- Story component understanding
- Sequencing
- Story review
- Expressive language

## Avocado Baby

By John Burningham

**Curriculum links**

- SEAL/PHSE – say no to bullying / healthy eating / relationships

- Narrative unit – stories in familiar setting / stories by the same author

- Science – heavy and light / weak and strong

- Topics – all about me / babies / food

## *Session 1*

### Introduction

*Sit around the story square.*

Recap on group rules:

Introduce story and basics of story, including being strong and saying 'no' to bullies.

Describe how session will run and content of session.

Developing:
- Understanding group rules
- Familiarity of story

## Warm up

### *Heavy or light*

The children should find a space in the room – first practice what they would look like picking something light up. . . . the vocabulary around this: easy / happy / relaxed / quick.

Then practice what they would look like picking something heavy up . . . the vocabulary around this: struggle / slow / annoyed / out of breath.

Developing:

- Attention and Listening
- Vocabulary
- Categorising
- Processing
- Concepts: heavy & light

The practitioner then shouts out different items to the children, and they have to pretend to pick them up, thinking about whether the item is heavy or light – for example:

Elephant / car / lorry / skip / tree / lion / house / bear / bench / table

Feather / paper / pencil / book / shoe / t-shirt / ball / spoon / cup

## Focus one

### *Bullying opinions*

This is an activity based on an activity found in *Learning through Drama in the Primary Years* (Farmer, 2012).

One side of the room should have a 'tick' symbol (standing for 'agree'), and the other side of the room should have a 'cross' symbol (standing for 'disagree').

Read out one statement at a time (examples of some statements are below), and ask the children to place themselves according to what they think.

Developing:

- Attention
- Verbal reasoning
- Comprehension
- Language around bullying
- Inference
- Expressive Language

The children can stand in the middle if they are unsure or think it's a bit of both . . . they can be reminded that answers don't have to be one or the other.

The children can be encouraged to discuss their decisions with each other, and they can be asked to explain why they have chosen their particular location.

Following this, they can change position if they have formed a new opinion. (Define the word 'opinion' for the children and explain its meaning.)

Children may be at different levels . . . different levels of questions can be used here to differentiate.

## Basic

Show them a picture of a well-known bully character (like the troll / Rumpelstiltskin / wicked stepmother / Little Rabbit Foo Foo . . . etc.), and ask the child: Is this character a bully?

## More complex

Make a statement and see if they agree or disagree:

When a child is bullied, the child feels sad.

Bullies are very mean all the time.

## Higher-level reasoning and language

- It's best to keep it a secret if you are bullied.

- If you see somebody in trouble, you should try to stop the bullies.

- It's OK to call someone a name if you are only joking.

- It's better to tell a friend about bullying than to tell the teacher.

- If you ignore bullies, they will go away.

- Anyone can be a bully.

## Focus two

*Story square*

Acting out 'Avocado Baby' . . .

This story has speaking parts so children can copy the lines from the book as they are read.

## Completion

*Sit around story square.*

Recap and review:

> Story components 'Avocado Baby' – go through: who, where, when, what happened, problem, the end.
>
> Shower off session and de-roll.

Developing:

- Attention and Listening
- Story understanding
- Narrative development
- Processing
- Spoken language recall
- Social Skills (eye contact/ communication with others/ sharing space & cooperation/ NVC.

Developing:

- Story component understanding
- Sequencing
- Story review
- Expressive language

## Jack and the Beanstalk

By Benjamin Tabart

**Curriculum links**

- SEAL /PHSE – relationships

- Narrative unit – traditional and fairy stories

- Science – plants and growth

- Geography – wealth and poverty across the world

- Topics – explorers / once upon a time / castles / adventures

## Session 1

### Introduction

*Sit around the story square.*

Recap on group rules:

Introduce story and any knowledge the children have about 'Jack and the Beanstalk.'

Read half the story up to the beans being thrown out of the window.

Describe how session will run and content of session.

> Developing:
> - Understanding group rules
> - Familiarity of story

## Warm up

### *Sleeping giant*

Children sit in a circle. . . . One child is the Giant pretending to sleep with a bunch of keys nearby (ask the children what noises the giant may make sleeping: snores, grunts, talking in sleep, mumbles, heavy breathing etc.).

> Developing:
> - Attention and Listening
> - Vocabulary

The children are to re-act Jack stealing from the giant.

The Giant has to listen with eyes closed. The Giant keeps his eyes closed (or use a blindfold), and, if he hears a sound, he points to the direction of where the sound comes from . . . if he points directly at Jack, then Jack has to sit down, and it is another child's turn.

The child chosen from the circle has to sneak around the Giant and grab the keys without the Giant hearing and not get pointed at directly.

## Focus one

### *Character game*

Discuss characters in the story: emphasise the 'who' component.

Help the children generate vocabulary linked to characters . . . encourage synonyms:

Giant:   Big . . . huge . . . gigantic . . .
         fierce . . . ferocious . . .
         aggressive
Jack:    Small . . . little . . . tiny
         Lazy . . . idol . . . slow moving
Mother:  Angry . . . annoyed . . . cross
Cow:     Sad . . . upset . . . unhappy . . . miserable

Developing:
- Attention and listening
- Vocabulary
- Line/ language rehearsal
- 'Who' component

The children walk around the room as each character showing the characteristics discussed. . . . Use this time to repeat and model vocabulary to them as they are acting.

Make the game quicker, and introduce a listening element:

Shout out a character and then shout out another . . . and so on. . . . The children have to listen and change character as soon as they hear the label.

Extension: introduce an appropriate phrase or word they should use while acting out the character. The children can generate this, or, if it is too difficult, the practitioner can give them the phrase. . . .

Giant: 'Fee Fi Fo Fum.'

Jack: 'Wow a Beanstalk!'

Mother: "Go to bed without any supper!"

Cow: 'Moo.'

## Focus two

### Market scene

Have one child as Jack and one child as the cow.

Get others to then spread around room and pretend to have a market stall (two children can share a market stall).

Developing:
- Attention
- Vocabulary/ categorisation
- Social skills: turn taking/ conversation skills
- 'Where' component

Ask the children what their stall is and what they are selling, or delegate them a stall:

The children are to generate appropriate vocabulary and category: fruit, vegetables, clothes, shoes, jewellery, house items etc.

Move on to the children then creating the market scene – shout out what they are selling:

'Come and get your oranges – fresh juicy oranges.'

Encourage children who don't want to do this to make sound effects using their voices or their bodies (rustling, stamping, etc.).

Jack is to walk round with his cow and make conversation with the market sellers – ask what they are selling and ask them if they want to buy his cow. . . .

## Completion

### Sit around story square.

Recap and review:

> Story components Jack and the
> Beanstalk go through: who, where,
> when, problem.
>
> Predict what may happen next.
>
> Shower off session and de-roll.

Developing:
- Story component understanding
- Prediction/inference
- Story review
- Expressive language

## Session 2

### Introduction

### Sit around the story square

Recap on group rules:

Recap story so far of 'Jack and the Beanstalk': who, where, when, problem.

Developing:
- Understanding group rules
- Familiarity of story

Describe how session will run and content of session.

## Warm up

### Beans game

The children come up with different types of beans – with help if needed – and then name and do an action with each bean (jumping beans: jump on the spot / runner beans: run on the spot / baked beans: get into tiny squashed up ball in a tin / broad beans: stretch out wide / jelly beans: wobble on the spot).

Developing:
- Attention and Listening
- Vocabulary (beans/verbs)

The children walk around the room and stop when the practitioner says 'freeze' – the practitioner shouts out a bean for the children to act out . . . can speed it up and go from one to another 'broad bean . . . baked bean . . . jelly bean!'

## Focus one

### Growing beanstalks

The children start as a seed and curl up small on the floor.

Generate synonyms for small (tiny/miniscule/incy-wincy/weeny).

The children pretend they are the beanstalk and they grow and become big.

Developing:
- Attention
- Vocabulary (describing)

Generate synonyms for big (huge/ginormous/massive/humungous).

The practitioner is to narrate and use the words the children have generated as they are seeds and then slowly grow.

## Focus two

### Conscience alley

This is an approach for exploring any kind of dilemma faced by a character.

The group forms two lines facing each other. One child walks between the lines as each member of the group speaks (or whispers – but loud enough to hear) his or her advice. When the character reaches the end of the alley, he or she makes a decision.

Lines can be arranged so that those on one side give opposing advice to those on the other.

In this story the decision process can be whether Jack should steal the items and/or whether he should go back up the beanstalk to the castle again. . . .

Developing:

- Attention
- Verbal Reasoning Skills
- Prediction
- Processing
- Memory
- Expressive Language Skills

The children should generate answers to why he should and why he shouldn't, then Jack walks down the alley . . . and states his decision once he gets to the end.

The child playing Jack can also state which piece of advice persuaded him or her the most.

This is an opportunity to discuss: what is fair and unfair, and what is right and wrong?

## Completion

*Sit around story square.*

Recap and review:

Developing:

- Story component understanding
- Sequencing
- Story review
- Expressive language

Story components 'Jack and the Beanstalk' go through: who, where, when, problem, what happened, the end.

Shake off session and de-roll.

## Additional or alternative activities

*Mantle of the Expert*

The children are in role as expert advisors.

The teacher is in role as Jack: explains the situation to the children and how Jack feels. . . .

Situation: Jack wants to make amends with the giant because the giant is actually kind and now has no money because his things were stolen from him.

Discuss: How can Jack show the giant he is sorry? Get together as a super-helper group and find a way to advise. . . .

Developing:
- Attention
- Problem solving skills
- Verbal reasoning
- Sequencing
- Social skills; negotiation/ conversation/ cohesion
- Expressive Language

Could it be that they:

- produce a sorry letter (verbally or written or both)?

- create a party in the village – produce a list of what they will need and how to invite the giant?

- give him his things back but ask him to share some of it so that Jack and the villagers can have some of the money too, so they can afford to eat and stay warm – produce a rota or way of sharing?

Extension: act out the scenario produced and what happens next.

## Story square

Acting out 'Jack and the Beanstalk'

. . .

This story has speaking parts so children can copy the lines from the book as they are read.

Developing:
- Attention and Listening
- Story understanding
- Narrative development
- Processing
- Spoken language recall
- Social Skills (eye contact/ communication with others/ sharing space & Co-operation/ NVC

# Child's own story

## *Collection*

Find a quiet space and explain to the child that it is his or her turn to make up his or her very own story. Have a prompt sheet and present this to the child so that the child can easily see it. This can help the child remember the story components and use them to create the story.[1]

The person writing the story writes down the child's response verbatim . . . if the child makes grammatical errors, then model back the sentence to him or her and write it down in its correct form. (This is to help the child reflect on the appropriate use of language, and other children will be exposed to this story so it is appropriate that other children hear the correct language and grammar use.)

The prompt sheet also has a box at the end labelled 'describe.' The person taking down the story can point to the 'describe' box to prompt the child to put a describing word before a word he or she may have used.

For example:

| | |
|---|---|
| *Child:* | 'The witch shouted "I'm going to cast a spell on you." ' |
| *Practitioner:* | (points *to describe box*) 'Can you put a describing word before "witch"?' |
| *Child:* | 'The angry witch!' |

\* Be aware of a balance with this, and do not interrupt story flow too many times. Do what is appropriate for the child and the flow of the story.

The practitioner can also prompt in places where a character may say something but the child has not stated any dialogue: 'What did they say?'

For example:

| | |
|---|---|
| *Child:* | 'The ninja found the treasure and took it back to his master.' |
| *Practitioner:* | 'What did the master say?' |
| *Child:* | 'He said, "Thank-you brave warrior"!' |
| *Practitioner writes:* | *The ninja found the treasure and took it back to his master.* |
| | *The master said, 'Thank-you brave warrior.'* |

As the child goes through the story, the practitioner can point to the story components on the prompt card to help guide the child to use them if needed.

Ask the child for a title to the story.

Create a session around the theme of the story with an appropriate warm up, focus, and story square.

*This activity develops children's ability to create their own stories using story language, sequencing, and describing vocabulary. They may base their stories on one they already know. . . .*

## Example session around a child's story

### 'Dinosaurs'

By Rafferty Lea-Trowman

Once upon a time there lived people and dinosaurs and the people (maked) made a dinosaur called Indominous Rex.

The scary, mean Indominous Rex escaped. The people got weapons and tried to catch it and they got the T-Rex to get it. Then the fast Raptors jumped on the Indominous Rex and at the end the massive dinosaur from the water jumped on the Indominous Rex and got him.

Then the T-Rex said 'thank-you' to the Raptors.

Then the mum came and the kids were safe and she said 'You're ok!'

The End

## Introduction

*Sit around the story square.*

Recap on group rules:

Introduce the title of the story from the child.

Read the story out loud to everyone.

Describe how session will run and content of session.

Developing:
- Understanding group rules
- Familiarity of story

## Warm up

### Dinosaur egg

Get an egg, make an egg, rugby ball etc.

All the children sit in a group, and one person is chosen to be the dinosaur. The chosen person must face away from the group and place the dinosaur egg behind himself or herself. One of the children will steal the egg and sit back down. The child can hide the egg behind his or her back or between his or her legs. Once it is hidden all the children say together:

'Dino, Dino, look around,

Your egg has gone, can it be found?'

Then the dinosaur must try to guess who stole the egg. If the dinosaur guesses right, the child gets to be the dinosaur again. If the child guesses incorrectly, the person who stole the egg gets to be the next dinosaur. . . . Play and repeat. . . .

Extend: the child who is the dinosaur labels the kind of dinosaur he or she is: T-Rex, Raptor, Stegosaurus, Triceratops etc.

> Developing:
> - Attention
> - Eye contact
> - Turn taking

## Focus one

### Palaeontologists

The children are put into small groups. They are given a scenario:

They are *palaeontologists* – discuss the meaning of this word. They need to find a bone, and once they have found it they need to investigate what kind of dinosaur it might have been.

> Developing:
> - Attention
> - Social Skills; cohesion/ negotiation/ turn taking/ tolerance
> - Inference
> - Prediction
> - Dinosaur related vocabulary

First they need to pack a bag of things they need to take with them on an *expedition* . . . and work together to come up with what they are going to take.

The practitioner cuts out bone shapes from paper and hides them around the room.

Each group is given instructions to follow to find that bone – for example: 'Go to the end of the room, turn left, and look somewhere where you might hear music' (under the piano at the end of the hall).

They are then asked to look at the bone and decide: Was it a big or small dinosaur? What might it have eaten? Did it have enemies? How did it become *extinct*? What name can you give it? Make one up, or use one you know.

The practitioner can give these questions for them to answer and work on together.

At the end, the children present to the other groups their bone and the facts they have come up with.

## Focus two

### *Story square*

Acting out 'Dinosaurs' story . . .

Developing:
- Story Square Skills

## Completion

### *Sit around the story square.*

Go over story components from child's story: who, where, when, problem, what happened, the end.

Developing:
- Story component understanding
- Expressive language
- Giving and receiving peer feedback

Each child is to say something that he or she likes about the story or the session.

Shake off the session and de-roll.

## Note

1  See Appendix E for prompt sheet.

# Chapter four
# KEY STAGE 2

The following section of this programme focuses on Key Stage 2.

Topics and stories found in this key stage provide ideas for enhancing knowledge and language of story/topic.

(The sessions are more suited to Years 3 and 4; however, this is dependent on the language and learning levels of the children participating.)

The following sessions are structured differently from the Key Stage 1 section. They are not written as specific session plans but provide different activities that can be used and chosen as appropriate by the practitioner to suit that week's learning/story/chapter.

Many of the ideas and activities can be used in other stories and topics with just the content within the activity changed.

Romans and Ancient Egypt are two topics chosen in this book to show how activities can be designed around topics such as these. There are obviously many topics covered at Key Stage 2; however, these should show ranges of activities and what they work on.

Many of the activities can be changed to suit different topics.

## George's Marvellous Medicine
By Roald Dahl

### Curriculum links

- SEAL/PHSE – relationships / say 'no' to bullying / changes

- Narrative unit – significant authors

- General themes: growing up / perseverance / dysfunctional families / putting right to a wrong . . .

*This book is significantly longer and more complex than those used in the Key Stage 1 section.*

*The story cannot be read or covered in one or two sessions.*

*Sessions can be run chapter by chapter so it is only one or two chapters read in the story square each session.*

*These sessions can be used to pre-teach and/or support the story that is being studied in the classroom or used as a story to work on over a series of sessions to encourage language and communication skills.*

## Introduction

Sit around the story square.

Go over group rules.

Use story component cards to recap elements of the story – adding in solution: who, where, when, the problem, what happened, the solution, the end.

Go over session content and how it will run.

### Objectives

For children to recap on group rules and respect for each other within a group context.

To recap on main elements of story/topic they are covering.

To be briefed on the session content and expectation.

## Warm ups

Choose from a selection of warm ups from the warm-up section.

## Specific warm ups for 'George's Marvellous Medicine'

### Vocabulary walk

Everyone lists the animals that appear in the book: Hen, Pig, Pony, Sheep, Goat, Bullock. What do they look like, how do they present, and what noise do they make?

Walk around the room, and then, when the practitioner shouts out an animal, the children have to act the animal out . . . you can go from one animal to another quickly ('Pony . . . hen . . . goat! Everyone walking again').

Children can also be out if they are last into their animal position.

Alternatively, the same activity can be used around verbs in the book:

grow, shrink, explode, drink, stir etc.

> Developing: attention and listening / vocabulary from book / processing

## Alliteration names extension

This is similar to the activity in the warm-up section; however, rather than the described activity, change it so that each child should come up with the same first sound, and each child should come up with a title of a made-up book similar to George's Marvellous Medicine – for example:

'Beth's Amazing Animals'

'Emma's Fantastic Foxes'

'Finn's Roaring Rockets' . . . and so on.

Once the child has completed his or her name alliteration, everyone copies it verbatim all together – e.g. Frank: 'Frank's dangerous dinosaur' . . . everyone repeats 'Frank's dangerous dinosaur.'

> Developing: attention and listening / phonological awareness: initial sound / alliteration knowledge and use / processing and imitation

## Grandma's footsteps

One child is Grandma and faces the wall. The others in the group start at the other end of the room, then try to creep up to Grandma and tap her on the shoulder. However, at any moment, Grandma can turn around suddenly. If she sees anyone moving, she points at them, and that person must return to the start. Nobody can move while she is watching them.

Whoever manages to tap her on the shoulder becomes Grandma, and the game starts again.

> Developing: attention and listening

## Focus activities

### Story square

Acting out chapters of 'George's Marvellous Medicine' . . .

This story has speaking parts so children can copy the lines from the book as they are read.

Some dialogue between two characters can be long. . . . Remember to 'whoosh' fairly regularly to keep all children involved and interactive. Remember to put inanimate items into the square (door, shed, house) and other characters: animals.

> Developing: attention and listening / story understanding / narrative development / processing / comprehension / spoken language recall / social skills (eye contact / communication with others / sharing space and cooperation / non-verbal communication)

### Verb or noun

There are many nouns and verbs in this book, and it is full of vocabulary. This activity works on discrimination of nouns and verbs:

Put the word 'NOUN' on a piece of paper on one side of the room and 'VERB' on the other.

All children stand in centre of the room. The practitioner reads out a noun or verb from the book, and children run to the correct side.

Extend: the children can add a describing word to the word that has been read out (child chosen randomly) – e.g. 'shampoo' . . . the child chosen gives the describing word 'shiny shampoo.'

Nouns from the story: George, Grandma, Pig, Pony, Bullock, Mrs Kranky, bottle, shampoo, saucepan, shed, kitchen, chicken, egg, pumpkin seed, roof, chair.

Verbs: drink, lie, glared, peck, shout, watch, tipped, sloshed, squawked, fly, discovered, open, emptied, jump, lowered, grew, blew, cackled, towering, look, ran, flapped.

Extension: make it more difficult by discriminating between verbs and adjectives, or adverbs and adjectives . . .

Developing: attention and listening / vocabulary categorising / book-specific vocabulary / use of describing vocabulary

## Guess the noun

Read out a passage from the book. . . . Everyone should find a space and act out the story as the practitioner reads it. The practitioner will subtract a word (noun), and the children together or individually chosen have to complete the missing word – e.g. George sat himself down at the . . .

Developing: attention and listening / comprehension / processing / noun awareness / inference

## Medicine walk

Re-create the scene where George goes around the house making the medicine. However, the children are to name their own items as they pretend to go into different rooms.

The practitioner should emphasise that this is about *where* George goes . . .

The practitioner starts the walk off, and the children follow.

The practitioner will narrate: 'First we are in the kitchen, and we grab a saucepan.' . . . The children pretend to grab a saucepan and carry it. 'Now let's start where George starts and go upstairs to the bathroom.'

Everyone follows the practitioner and pretends to climb the stairs and enter the bathroom. Ask each child to name an item that he or she is putting in the saucepan. Encourage an appropriate item that would be found in a bathroom.

Once everyone has labelled an item, the practitioner moves on: 'OK, let's move into the bedroom.' Continue as before with the children naming an item, and then move into the laundry room, then back to the kitchen, then out to the shed, then to the garage and back to the kitchen to turn on the stove.

Extension: have the children say what the item they have listed will do with a rehearsed scaffolded sentence – for example:

'I'm putting in . . . because it will make grandma clean.'

> Developing: attention and listening / vocabulary categorisation / sentence construction with 'because' conjunction / verbal reasoning / 'where' narrative component

## Punctuation game

Discuss punctuation with the children: question mark, exclamation mark, full stop.

Show them the three symbols[1] and give an example sentence to go with it.

Show them a written sentence example also.

Then hold each mark up, and show the children the sign to go with it:

Question mark: curve the hand around the top and down with a punch at the bottom for the dot.

Full stop: punch the hand forward.

Exclamation mark: bring the hand down in a line, and then punch forward to make the dot.

Read a piece of dialogue from the book slowly.

Firstly, hold the symbol up to the children when they should sign the punctuation – for example:

The practitioner reads 'It's time for my medicine!' and holds up the exclamation mark – all the children do the action of the exclamation mark at the end of the sentence. Continue with other punctuation.

To make it easier, get them to listen for and do action of one punctuation mark and introduce more punctuation as they improve.

Extension: remove the symbol prompts.

Further extension: introduce speech-marks into activity

Speech marks: raise the hands to the side of the head, and get two fingers out (index and middle) and bend and straighten them (this sign is often used by adults when they 'quote' something).

Developing: attention and listening / punctuation vocabulary and awareness / processing

## Making a medicine

Using the list of items in the book, the practitioner pretends there is a giant saucepan in the centre of the circle.

The practitioner facilitates the children generating a large selection of verbs for putting items in:

sprayed, squirted, chucked, poured, threw, added, tipped, squeezed, placed, sieved, sprinkled, scattered.

Each child takes turns to stand and put an item in.

As the child stands, the child should make a sentence with the item (noun) and the verb given to him or her by the practitioner – for example:

Words: 'squirted' and 'toothpaste'

Child: 'George squirted the toothpaste into the saucepan.'

Extension: to make it more difficult, give them the item only, so that they themselves have to generate an appropriate verb to go with it.

Further extension: have the child add a describing word into the sentence if possible:

'George squirted the *white sticky* toothpaste into the saucepan.'

Then all stand and mix the medicine in the enormous saucepan together. Each child takes a sip of the medicine, pulls a face, and gives a describing word for how it tastes: 'It tastes amazing!'

Get all the other children to repeat the describing word together – e.g. child: 'It tastes ghastly!' All together: 'Ghastly!'

> Developing: attention and listening / sentence formulation / planning / vocabulary extension / imitation / memory / facial expression / non-verbal communication

## George's decision alley

This is an approach for exploring any kind of dilemma faced by a character (e.g. Red Riding Hood to speak to the wolf or the moment the wicked queen gives Snow White the poison apple).

The group forms two lines facing each other. One person walks between the lines as each member of the group speaks (or whispers – but loud enough to hear) his or her advice. When the character reaches the end of the alley, she makes her decision.

The lines can be arranged so that those on one side give opposing advice to those on the other.

In this story the decision process can be whether to give Grandma the medicine or not. Children should generate answers to why he should and why he shouldn't – then George walks down the alley . . . and states his decision once he gets to the end.

The child playing George can also state which piece of advice persuaded him or her the most.

> Developing: verbal reasoning skills / prediction / processing / memory / expressive language skills

## Hot seat

Grandma is played by the practitioner. The other children ask questions to Grandma about her life.

Prepare the children to ask about different parts of her life and perhaps with the right questions so they can discover what made her so mean and horrible.

Prep the children before the activity, building their questioning by discussing and generating question words: who, where, when, how, why, what.

Extension: create a story piecing together the information from Hot Seating.

Develop the story and act it out in the story square.

Developing: attention and listening / question knowledge and use / comprehension / expressive language skills / story and narrative development

# Aesop's Fables

## *The Hare and the Tortoise*

### Curriculum links

- SEAL/PHSE – going for goals / getting on and falling out

- Narrative unit/topic – myths, legends, fables, traditional tales / Ancient Greece

- General themes – perseverance / fables / doing things fast doesn't mean well / putting effort in

## *The Lion and the Mouse*

### Curriculum links

- SEAL/PHSE – getting on and falling out / relationships / good to be me

- Narrative unit/topic – myths, legends, fables, traditional tales / Ancient Greece

- General themes – fables / helping others / friends

## Introduction

Sit around the story square.

Go over group rules.

Go over session content and how it will run.

Discuss what *Aesop's Fables* are. Use story components:

*Who*: Aesop was a writer. People say he was a slave who gained his freedom through the good advice he gave to his masters. However, it is not certain whether he actually existed at all, or whether he is simply a legendary person.

*Where*: from Ancient Greece.

*When*: thought to have lived around 600 BC.

*What*: he is said to have written a number of well-known fables. Fables are often through the image of animals who speak or otherwise take on human characteristics.

*The end*: fables generally give a moral message to think about.

## Objectives

For children to recap on group rules and respect for each other within a group context.

To recap on main elements of story/topic they are covering.

To be briefed on the session content and expectation.

## Warm ups

Choose from a selection of warm ups from the warm-up section.

### *Specific warm ups for Aesop's fables*

Hare and the tortoise race

The participants are asked to 'race' from one end of the room to the other. However, the race must be done in slow motion. Whoever can move the slowest is the winner!

## Animal game

The children walk around the room and act out the animal shouted out: hare / tortoise / lion / mouse.

Extend so that the children have to find a partner when the practitioner shouts 'stop' and then act out how a mouse and a lion or hare and tortoise would be together.

Developing: Attention and listening / social skills in paired work

## Hunter/lion/mouse

This is a stuck-in-the-mud-style game. . . . Two children are the hunters, and the other children are lions. The children run around the room . . . and the hunters have to tag ('trap') the lions.

If trapped, the child who is the lion has to go down to the floor and curl up (pretending to be in a net).

The child can be *freed/rescued* by another child by that child changing role quickly and pretending to be a mouse . . . crouching down and pretending to nibble before the hunter tags him or her.

Developing: attention / character vocabulary and story comprehension / group cohesion

# Focus activities

## *Story square*

Acting out the story of 'The Hare and the Tortoise' or 'The Lion and the Mouse' . . . These stories are short and easy to download from various Internet sources.

These stories have dialogue so children can copy the lines from the book as they are read.

> Developing: attention and listening / story understanding / narrative development / processing / comprehension / spoken language recall / social skills (eye contact / communication with others / sharing space and cooperation / non-verbal communication)

## Fable animals

Think of some animals and how in fables they are given stereotypical human characteristics: explain the word 'stereotype' with examples.

The children are to use their bodies and then describe how they have presented themselves to show that characteristic – for example:

'A lion is brave' – everyone use their bodies to show 'brave.' The child chosen should describe what her or she has done: 'I have made myself big and have stuck my chest out.'

'A squirrel is shy' – everyone use their bodies to show 'shy.' The child chosen should describe what he or she has done: 'I have made myself small and I'm hiding my face.'

Other examples: 'Foxes are sly,' 'Ants are hardworking' . . . etc.

## Vocabulary run

Have a picture or written word on each side of the room: one with 'tortoise' and one with 'hare.'

The children stand in the middle of the room. The practitioner reads out vocabulary that is related to either the tortoise or the lion. The children run to the side of the room they think belongs with that word.

Vocabulary to use:

loud / quiet / slow / steady / sensible / careful / silly / show off / clever / boastful / winner.

Once the practitioner has modelled vocabulary, other children can take the practitioner role and shout out vocabulary for the group.

The same game can be played with 'The Lion and the Mouse' story. One side of the room is 'mouse,' and the other side is 'lion.'

Extension: this time, vocabulary is more ambiguous and not as exact and could apply to either character. Explain this to the children.

Once they have gone to the character they think the word belongs to, ask each child why he or she made his or her decision so that the child explains his or her choice – for example:

> 'Lewis, the word was "brave" . . . why did you choose the lion side?' Lewis may say, 'Because lions are brave.' The practitioner agrees: 'Yes, well done. . . . Sophia, why did you choose the mouse?' Sophia: 'Because the mouse was brave to stay and nibble through the net.' The practitioner agrees: 'Yes – so both answers are correct because you explained your opinions.'

Vocabulary to use: big / little / squeak / roar / laugh / kind / brave / scared / helpful / friend / trapped

Developing: attention and listening / processing / vocabulary understanding and use / verbal reasoning / inference / expressive language – use of 'because' to answer a question

## Television interview

The practitioner facilitates discussion around what an *interview* is and how they work. Have the children seen interviews on TV?

Generate questions they might ask the Tortoise, the Hare and the Lion. They could pretend they are at the Olympics for the Hare and Tortoise interviews and pretend the Lion is on a rescue programme.

Have the children get into groups of three. Each child is given a role of either Character, Interviewer or Cameraperson.

Each child has a job:

Interviewer – to ask the character questions

Character – to answer the questions

Cameraperson – to tell the characters where to stand and to pretend to film them . . . they must say 'action' and 'that's a wrap!'

The activity can be rotated three times so each child gets a turn at being the Character, Interviewer and Cameraperson.

Less-able children can do the Cameraperson role, whilst more-able children can do the Interviewer or Character roles.

## Make own fable

The practitioner facilitates the group making its own fable.

Sit around the story square and go around to each child asking them questions to build up a story with their answers.

Tips for creating a fable to give children before they start:

> Create characters that are simple stereotypes rather than complicated heroes or villains. Make the main characters animals, and have them behave like human stereotypes: E.g. a wise old turtle, a cunning fox, a lazy donkey.

Use the names of the main characters to give the fable a title: 'The Fox and the Bird.'

State the moral of the fable before the story starts so they know where they are heading.

Keep description to a minimum, and use dialogue only to help tell what happens.

Use story components to help make the start simple: . . . Once . . . there was a . . . who lived in . . .

Once the story is complete, the practitioner puts it together, and it is acted out in the story square.

Developing: Attention and listening / processing and comprehension / narrative structure / expressive language / use of conjunctions to link each other's parts of the story / inference and prediction

## Where The Wild Things Are
By Maurice Sendak

Although this story is not complex and can be read in one sitting easily, it has excellent content and opportunities to explore ideas introduced in the story at a higher level.

Again these activity ideas could be transferred to other stories the children are covering and are not only achievable with this story.

### Curriculum links

- SEAL/PHSE – new beginnings / relationships / good to be me

- Narrative unit/topic – fantasy / explorers / philosophy

- General themes – travel / mischief / punishment / imagination / creating new worlds

## *Introduction*

Sit around the story square.

Go over group rules.

Go over session content and how it will run.

Discuss the story 'Where the Wild Things Are.'

What do children know about it already?

Read the story.

Ask some philosophical questions – children don't need to answer them now, but, perhaps after doing some sessions, process the drama together.

*Questions for philosophical discussion*

- How does Max feel when his mother sends him to his room?

- Do you think that Max's punishment is fair? Why or why not?

- Is there a different punishment that would have been better?

- Should parents punish their children? Why or why not?

- Where are the wild things?

- Do you think the wild things are real?

- Did Max dream them? Imagine them?

- What's the difference between real things and dreams?

- Can you tell that you are not dreaming now?

- Have you ever felt loved best of all by someone?

- Have you ever felt that no one loved you best of all?

- Why is it important to feel loved best of all?

## Objectives

For children to recap on group rules and respect for each other within a group context.

To recap on main elements of story/topic they are covering.

To be briefed on the session content and expectation.

Preparation: to start thinking about questions that can be answered after some drama and language work.

## *Warm ups*

Choose a warm up from the warm-up section.

## Specific warm ups for 'Where the Wild Things Are'

### Role-play to music

Put on music and ask children to make mischief like Max (but make it in slow motion, and remind them to make movements slow and big).

Stop the music and have the children freeze in their current pose.

Developing: attention / imagination / non-verbal communication

### The wild rumpus

Everyone begin frozen in a rumpus shape – discuss what 'rumpus' means and other words for this. A child is designated as Max and shouts, 'Let the wild rumpus begin!' Then the music and rumpus begins. When Max yells 'Stop!' the rumpus ends, music stops, and all freeze.

Developing: attention and listening / vocabulary synonyms

### Character cross-over greeting

The children line up in two lines facing each other. They think about what kind of wild thing they are going to be (encourage them to think about size, movement, facial expression, mood).

Then, when the practitioner says 'Go,' the children walk towards each other as their 'wild thing.' As they cross over and go past each other, they must greet each other in some way using greeting language (hello / pleased to meet you / nice to see you / how are you? / etc.).

They then turn around and cross back over and say a different greeting. They turn around and cross over a final time using departure language (goodbye / see you soon / take care / catch you later / bye for now / etc.).

Developing: attention / non-verbal communication (eye contact / use of body / social greeting and leaving language)

## Focus activities

### *Dreams*

Tell the children to close their eyes and save an image from a dream, just one image (e.g. falling / floating in a river / being in dinosaur times . . .).

The practitioner is the conductor, and when the practitioner touches a child's shoulder (all have their eyes closed), the child is encouraged to say a sentence describing his or her dream image with some describing words put in (example to give them: 'I see a rainbow with a shiny and gleaming pit of gold at the end'). After this they should say it every time the practitioner touches their shoulders.

Developing: attention / visualising / expressive language

### *Hot seat*

Mum is to be in the hot seat – three children could play Mum and take turns answering questions. The other children ask the questions.

Prepare the children to ask, what did Max do? How did Mum feel? What other punishments does she give Max if he is naughty? What did she make for his supper? Has Max got brothers and sisters? Are they naughty sometimes? Are there any other questions the children want to ask?

Developing: attention / asking questions / expressive language

## Max's alley

The children become 'wild things' facing each other in two lines with space between as an alleyway for the child who is playing 'Max' to walk. As the child walks down the alley, the children become 'wild things.'

Ask the children, how can they make themselves into wild things? For example: roll my eyes, show my terrible yellow teeth, grunt, howl, bang my chest . . .

The children are to say something to Max for coming to their island. Each child is given a word that he or she has to use in his or her sentence (e.g. given the word 'and,' the child says, 'Turn around *and* leave Max'; or given the word 'because,' the child says, 'We want you to stay *because* you are cool!'; or given the word 'strangers,' the child says, 'We don't want strangers on our island!') . . .

The wild things only say something when Max passes them, and they may not touch Max. They go silent when Max turns and says, 'Silent!'

Developing: attention / non-verbal communication / sentence formulation and planning

## *Imagination door*

The practitioner encourages the children to think of an imaginary world that is waiting for the children as they walk through their imaginary door. The children open an imaginary door in front of everyone else. They step through and act out what they can see . . . and the practitioner encourages them to ask each other questions such as, what does it look like? How does it smell? Who lives there? How do they feel?

Once a scene is set up, all the children stand up, and they open and step through their own doors into the first child's imaginary world. The practitioner provides a narrative for all the children to follow and asks individual children questions along the way:

'Everyone look into the sky . . . what can you see, Angelina? As you are walking, you trip . . . what did you just trip over, Alec? Everyone bend over and pick up the flower in front of you . . . Hugo how does it smell? Ruby how does it look? Now you have found a lake . . . Elliot can you describe how the lake looks? There is a boat . . . everyone get in . . . Stella, what is the weather like as you cross? Now we are at the other side . . . . Hugo what can you see?'

Developing: attention and listening / asking questions / comprehension / processing / expressive language and description skills

## Story square

Acting out the story of 'Where the Wild Things Are' . . .

This story has dialogue so children can copy the lines from the book as they are read.

You could also encourage some ad-libbing here and encourage children to make up dialogue with each other when they are in the story square as there are opportunities for this.

> Developing: attention and listening / story understanding / narrative development / processing / comprehension / spoken language recall / expressive language / social skills (eye contact / communication with others / sharing space and cooperation / non-verbal communication)

## Five things . . .

Ask the children: If they were going away for a year and a day, what five important things would they bring?

The children list their five things (can be verbal, written down, or drawn pictures) and then get into pairs . . . and they compare their lists and complete one list of five items between them, considering each other's items and explaining why they are important.

That pair then joins another pair, and again they compare lists and make a joint list. . . . Continue until the whole group has only one list.

> Developing: social skills (eye contact / turn taking / negotiation / verbal reasoning / use of 'because' / expressive language)

## TV trailer

Discuss what film trailers look like . . . have they seen one in the cinema or on the television? What do trailers show? Present vocabulary such as 'promote,' 'sell,' 'anticipate' and 'cliff-hanger.' Show the children a trailer if possible.

The children are to think about the main parts of the story that should be in a trailer:

Introduce Max

Mischief

Sails away

'Where the Wild Things Are'

The wild things

Make a cliff-hanger. . . . Will Max stay on the island forever? Are the wild things happy or angry? Is Max safe?

Storyboard this in diagram form for the children on a whiteboard/flipchart before they go off in groups so they have the sequence clearly mapped in their minds

The children should then split into groups and role-play a trailer of 'Where the Wild Things Are' in sequence. . . . Get one child to narrate the trailer as it is being acted.

Developing: attention / sequencing / non-verbal communication / social skills (turn taking / negotiation / eye contact / group cohesion / expressive language skills)

## Philosophical questions

Have the children answer some of the philosophical questions posed in the introduction.

Developing: higher-level thinking and language skills (reasoning / prediction / inference)

# Topic: the Romans

## Introduction

Sit around the story square.

Go over group rules.

Go over session content and how it will run.

Discuss the Romans – what do the children know about them already?

Use story components to guide questions:

Who were the Romans? What are the types of Romans or characters from stories they know that were Roman?

Where did they live?

When were the Romans around?

What did they do?

How many years did they last before their rule came to an end?

It would be useful to have pictorial support here and show children pictures of different Romans, where they lived on a map, what they did etc.[2]

## Objectives

For children to recap on group rules and respect for each other within a group context.

To introduce main elements of topic they are covering.

To be briefed on the session content and expectations.

## *Warm ups*

Choose from a selection of warm ups in the warm-up section.

## Specific warm ups for Romans

### *Centurion says . . .*

Explain to the children that a 'Centurion' is a leader of a large group of Roman soldiers in the army. Show a picture if possible.

Play the game similar to 'Simon Says.' Give instructions for the children to follow . . . if the Centurion doesn't say and the children still carry out the instruction, then they are out.

For example: 'Centurion says put your hands on your head.'

'Centurion says turn all the way around and count to 5.'

'Touch your toes and give someone a high-five.' . . . Anyone that carries out this task is out.

The centurion says to the child who is out: 'Roman soldier, you are dismissed!'

> Developing: attention and listening / introduction to Roman vocabulary / 'who' component

## I went to the Forum and bought . . .

Explain that a Forum was one of the important centres of Roman daily life. It was a big, open market area, surrounded by Roman banks, temples, baths, and businesses.

Play a game similar to the shopping game. . . . Ask the children to think of Roman items: 'I went to the Forum and bought . . . grapes / candles / lamp oil / dates / honey / a goat / jewellery / bread / a toga / sandals / fish / vegetables.'

Each child should try to remember what has been said before and come up with his or her own . . . see how far around the story square they can get.

> Developing: attention and listening / memory / topic vocabulary / 'where' component

## Months of the year line-up

Each child is given a month of the year written down on a piece of paper (with an image also if needed). The child holds this out so everyone can see.

Firstly, get all the children to chant the months of the year . . . and then explain that it was the Romans that created the calendar (e.g. July named after Julius Caesar).

The aim of the activity is for the children to work together and put themselves in order of the calendar: January through December. They are not allowed to talk or touch each other, so they have to work with their non-verbals.

Aim: for the children to be lined up January to December at the end of the activity.

(If there are less than 12 children, get adults to also hold up a month, or do it in two lots of six months. . . . If there are more than 12 children, get some children to be observers and watch behaviours and report back at the end.)

Developing: attention / social skills (turn taking / collaboration / tolerance / patience / eye contact / non-verbal communication / group cohesion) / months of the year vocabulary and sequence / 'when' component

## Months-of-the-year march

The practitioner stands at one end of the room, and all children stand in a line next to the practitioner with backs against the wall. The practitioner then starts marching forwards while saying the months of the year – and encouraging the children to join in.

The children have to march and stay in line with the practitioner.

The practitioner will shout 'stop' at some point and stop marching immediately . . . and the children have to try to stop with the practitioner.

Those children that step forwards and are out of line have to go back to the wall and march from there. . . . This repeats until some children get to the other side of the room with the practitioner.

Emphasise the word 'when' with the story component card. . . . Explain the months of the year and the link to the Romans.

Developing: attention and listening / months of the year vocabulary and sequencing / 'when' component

## Focus activities

## Roman character game

Discuss different types of Romans – emphasise and show the story component 'who.'

Help the children generate vocabulary linked to characters . . . and encourage synonyms.

Pictures to support the description would be useful here.

> Roman Soldier: brave . . . courageous . . . fearless . . . bold
>
> Gladiator: fierce . . . ferocious . . . aggressive
>
> Or if being made to fight: scared . . . terrified . . . helpless
>
> Emperor: powerful . . . important . . . commanding . . . ruler
>
> Servant:  sad . . . upset . . . unhappy . . . miserable . . . tired . . . exhausted . . . weary

Discuss how these characters would present: What might they wear or carry? What is their role/job?

Clothes vocabulary to use: helmet / body armour / shield / sword / spear / sandals / tunic (servants) / toga (emperor)

Get the children to walk around the room as each character, showing the characteristics discussed. . . . The practitioner uses this time to repeat and model vocabulary to them as they are acting. 'I can see some very important looking Emperors. . . . Ted looks like a powerful ruler with his head held high. . . .'

Make the game quicker and introduce a listening element: Shout out a character and then shout out another . . . and so on. . . . The children have to listen and change character as soon as they hear the name.

> Developing: attention and listening / processing / topic vocabulary / description vocabulary / 'who' component

## Roman gods character game

This game is similar to the previous Roman character game, but it introduces Roman gods – for example:

> Jupiter – King of the gods: most powerful god / rode a winged horse called Pegasus / his weapons were thunderbolts

> Neptune – God of the sea: very powerful / rode a dolphin or a horse / his weapon was a trident (three prongs) / his bad moods would affect the seas

> Diana – Goddess of the moon and of the hunt: cold and unfriendly / loved dogs / her weapon was a bow and arrow

Venus – Goddess of love and beauty: the myth says she was created from sea foam / she was beautiful / she represents water.

The children act out these gods when practitioner calls them out.

Developing: attention and listening / processing / topic vocabulary / description vocabulary / 'who' component

## Roman soundscapes

Discuss some different locations in Roman history and what sounds might be heard / what might be going on: emphasise the 'where' story component.

Have some pictures ready to show as you discuss and to support new vocabulary and ideas. Ask the children: How can we recreate these sounds? Extend and add to their answers:

Roman baths: water splashing / steam / people drying themselves / washing / people talking

Roman market (Forum): busy / people selling food / shouting out what they are selling / footsteps / money / horses hooves

Amphitheatres/Coliseum: shouting / cheering / clapping / booing / sound of swords / fighting / lions

Roman home: no TV . . . quiet / clinking of plates in kitchen / children playing / chickens in the garden / sweeping floors / banging rugs / washing clothes.

Once this has been discussed – one child leaves the room briefly, and the group are told what scene to create with just their voices and bodies. . . . A child comes into the room, closes his or her eyes, and listens to the scene that the group recreates and then guesses 'where' they are.

Different scenes can be created.

Developing: attention and listening / topic vocabulary / description vocabulary / 'where' component

## Story square

Acting out a story with Roman theme:

For example:

Romulus and Remus

Julius Caesar

Escape from Pompeii

Detectives in Togas

(many of these stories can be downloaded from the Internet)

Some of the focus activities listed can be changed to suit the 'who,' 'where' and 'when' elements of the Roman-themed story chosen to help embed the story further.

Developing: attention and listening / story understanding / narrative development / processing / comprehension / spoken language recall / expressive language / social skills (eye contact / communication with others / sharing space and cooperation / non-verbal communication)

## Roman towns

Discuss with the children how Romans built towns in Britain and created roads to connect these towns. Most places ending with 'chester,' 'caster' and 'cester' are most likely to be old Roman towns. . . .

Can the children name any places in the country with these endings?

Emphasise the 'where' component in this activity.

Play a differentiation game. The children walk around the room . . . it can be in the role as a type of Roman they choose (soldier, centurion, emperor, servant, gladiator, etc.)

The practitioner shouts out a place in the country. . . . If it has an ending that makes it an old Roman town, they stand up tall and stretch their arms out; if it is not, they crouch to the floor.

List of places with Roman endings: Manchester / Doncaster / Dorchester / Cirencester / Colchester / Leicester / Winchester / Worcester / Gloucester

Non-Roman endings: Nottingham / Sunderland / Liverpool / Swansea / Cardiff / Brighton / Birmingham / Newcastle

> Developing: attention and listening / processing / 'where' component / places vocabulary

## Roman numerals

Show the children the Roman numerals you want to work on (e.g. I, II, V, X). Go through the meaning of these and their corresponding number.

Then place a Roman numeral on each side of the room – so each side has a different numeral. The children are to stand in the middle. . . . The Practitioner shouts out a number, and the children run to its corresponding numeral.

> Developing: attention and listening / processing / memory / Roman numerals vocabulary / symbols

## Timeline pre-activity

This activity is to introduce CE and BCE vocabulary and the context of this within time.

Emphasise the 'when' component in this activity.

The children line up side by side and face a piece of string on the floor (or a line already there).

The space in front of the line stands for 'CE', which is 'Common Era' (this used to be better known as AD).

The space behind the line is 'BCE,' 'Before Common Era.'

The children are to listen out for 'Common Era' or 'CE,' and they jump over the line in front. When they hear 'BCE' or 'Before Common Era,' they jump behind the line.

This activity is similar to 'In the river, on the bank,' from 'The Three Billy Goats Gruff' session plan in this book. However, it is used in this activity to help visualise and experience time and its labels.

Developing: attention and listening / processing / 'when' component / era vocabulary

## Timeline

(It will be useful if children have participated in the timeline pre-activity before doing this so they are more familiar with 'CE' and 'BCE' terms.)

The children line up across the room to create a timeline (show them a diagram of a timeline to help them visualise this – this can be a Roman timeline or a simple timeline of their day.)

The children stand in the line – where the practitioner puts them.

Each child is given a role.

All have a practice at acting out their role all together, and adults help where needed.

Then the group stands in line quietly.

The practitioner will walk along the time line, and as the practitioner gets to each child, the child will shout out the date and the fact attached to that, and then the child acts it out. Once the practitioner moves on, the child stops and becomes still again.

This should look like a Mexican wave type effect with children only acting when the practitioner is next to them.

List for timeline:

Some of these can be taken out or others added depending on what the children are focusing on in lessons and what the main learning objective is in terms of time the children need to know. Some facts may be too complicated, and these can be removed.

(Vocabulary in italics will need explaining to children.)

753 BCE: building of Rome begins (the child should act out building and working).

510 BCE: *Officials* (*government*) are *elected* (*chosen*) to *rule* (*manage/run*) Rome (the child acts out looking important and ruling).

202 BCE: Rome *conquers* (*captures/takes*) areas outside Italy (the child acts out fighting and ruling).

130 BCE: Rome *conquers* the countries of Greece and Spain (the child acts out fighting and ruling).

55 BCE: Rome *invades* (*enters and takes*) Britain (the child acts out fighting and ruling).

CE 1: Jesus is born (the child acts out holding a baby / being a baby).

CE 61: *Boudicca* fights against the Romans: *Boudicca was the Queen of the East of England and fought against the Romans taking over and occupying Britain* (the child acts out being a queen and leading/fighting).

CE 122: the building of *Hadrian's Wall* began: *Hadrian's Wall was built to separate the North of Britain from the South to separate the Barbarians (people who were not seen as civilised and part of the Roman people) from the South and to create a border* (the child acts out building a wall or stretching himself or herself to look like a wall).

CE 200: Rome attacked by *Barbarians* (*not civilised / don't live like the Romans: don't use facilities like the Romans*) (the child acts out being a Barbarian or a Roman in battle).

CE 235–285: 20 Roman Emperors are *assassinated* (killed because they are a leader) (the child acts out being assassinated or assassinating).

CE 410: Romans *rule* of Britain ends, and they leave (the child acts marching away, waving off the soldiers etc.).

CE 455: Roman Empire *collapses* (*falls/ends*) (child acts out Soldiers falling, buildings falling etc.).

Developing: attention and listening / topic specific vocabulary / processing / comprehension / 'when' component / sequencing

## Hadrian's fact hunt

Discuss Hadrian's Wall and what it was:

Show the children a map if possible showing where the wall would have been.

Ask the children to go on a fact hunt. . . . Each child is given a fact – it can be written down to help them remember, or key words are given to help.

Each child goes around the room and finds another child. . . . They shake hands and tell each other their facts. Then they thank each other and move on.

At the end everyone comes together and has to tell everyone a fact they have remembered from their fact-finding activity.

At the end everyone should remember their own fact and one other.

Facts such as:

* Romans built a wall from one *coast* over to the other *coast* (from East to West).
* It was built to protect England from *tribes* in Scotland.
* The Emperor Hadrian ordered the wall to be built
* The wall allowed soldiers to *control* who came in and out.
* Every mile there was a *gateway* called *Mile castles.*
* Large *forts* were built along the wall.
* *Forts* could have up to 1,000 Roman Soldiers in them.
* The wall was about 84 *miles* long.

> Developing: attention and listening / processing / memory / comprehension / vocabulary / social skills (turn taking / eye contact / starting and finishing an interaction) / 'what' component

## Hadrian's Wall

The children all hold hands across the room and create 'Hadrian's Wall.'

One child from the end walks around to the middle of the line, and the two children in the middle let go of hands and create a 'gateway' or 'mile castle.'

The practitioner asks the child to name vocabulary items or answer a topic-related question. . . . If the child is correct, the child passes through the gateway and joins the other end of the line. (Try to match correct-level questions with the children and differentiate the questions asked for the different levels.)

Then the next child from the other end of the line comes round to the middle, and everyone shifts up one . . . etc.

The practitioner facilitates the movement of this activity and emphasises vocabulary as they narrate 'Hadrian's Wall / Gateway / Mile castle / East Coast side / West Coast side.

Question examples:

Name two kinds of Romans (Soldier, Emperor, Slave etc.).

Where did Romans go for entertainment?

Name a Roman god.

Name a Roman Emperor.

What is the name of the wall the Romans built to protect the south of Britain from the North?

Tell me something about Hadrian's Wall.

What are the months of the year?

Name an item of clothing that Romans wore.

Developing: attention / vocabulary and language recap / answering questions

## Topic: Ancient Egypt

### Introduction

Sit around the story square.

Go over group rules.

Go over session content and how it will run.

Discuss Ancient Egypt vs. Modern Egypt – what do children know about it already?

Use story components to guide questions:

Who were the Egyptians? Types of Egyptians or characters from stories they know that were Egyptian?

Where did Egyptians live, work etc.?

When were the Ancient Egyptians around?

What did they do?

It would be useful to have pictorial support here and show children pictures of different Egyptians, where Egypt is on a map, what they did etc.[3]

### Objectives

For children to recap on group rules and respect for each other within a group context.

To introduce main elements of topic they are covering.

To be briefed on the session content and expectation.

## Warm ups

Choose from a selection of warm ups from the warm-up section.

## Specific warm ups for Ancient Egypt

### Howard Carter's 'I spy'

Discuss who 'Howard Carter' is. If children are unsure / haven't covered this yet, then explain who he is:

the archaeologist who discovered Tutankhamen's (Pharaoh) tomb in 1922.

*Archaeology* is the study of things that people made, used, and left behind so we can understand what people of the past were like and how they lived. . . .

The practitioner tells the children that archaeologists are good at looking for things and 'spying things,' and everyone has to pretend to be Howard Carter on their turn. . . .

Every child on their turn will say, 'I'm Howard Carter . . . I spy with my little eye something beginning with . . .' and play the usual game of 'I spy.'

> Developing: attention / topic vocabulary introduction / phonological awareness: initial sound identification

## Egyptian ship

The children are to imagine they are on an Egyptian ship sailing down the river Nile.

As the children are sailing, the ship will go North / East / South / West. Four sides of the room should be labelled with these.

When one of the directions is called out, the children run to the appropriate side of the room. In-between shouting out these directions, the children should follow these instructions when the practitioner shouts them out:

'Row the boat!' – arms mime rowing with oars

'Pass a pyramid' – everyone put arms up into a pyramid shape

'Scrub the decks' – get down to the floor and mime scrubbing

'Land ahoy' – hand to brow as if searching and shout 'Ahoy!'

> Developing: attention and listening / processing / topic vocabulary and information

## Mummy team challenge

Children line up in two teams behind each other. They pass a balloon or ball between their legs to the person behind. When the ball gets to the last person, that person has to walk like a 'mummy' with the ball to the front and start the process again of passing ball through legs.

The winning team is the first team to get the starting team member back to the front again.

> Developing: attention and listening / group cohesion

## Across the Nile

The children make two lines facing each other and imagine they are standing on the banks of the 'Nile.'

One child is chosen to lead . . . and that child then chooses a child in one line. The first child stands behind the chosen child and asks chosen child to close his or her eyes and then gently pushes the chosen child so he or she sets sail across the 'Nile.'

The child with eyes closed walks slowly across the river. On the other side of the 'Nile,' the children should be ready to catch the child coming towards them.

When someone catches the child, the child can then open his or her eyes. . . . The child that caught the other child says 'Thank-you' to the child and then takes the place of the child that caught him or her.

He or she then gently pushes the other child across the line (the other side should all move along by one or two to make sure different children get turns).

Extend by adding two or three children crossing at once.

> Developing: attention / social skills (eye contact / trust)

## Musical Pharaohs

A game of musical statues . . . if possible, play the music 'Walk like an Egyptian' (by 'The Bangles' [1986]).

Show children the 'Egyptian walk' (one hand in front and one behind, and they push out and in). Get the children to walk/dance around like this and explain to the children the 'hieroglyphics' showed pictures of Egyptian people with their arms in this position and how it is believed they may have danced like this.

Play the music and stop it – everyone should freeze – anyone that moves is out.

(Explain the word 'hieroglyphics' and show them images if possible . . . get the children to say the word 'hieroglyphics' themselves.)

Developing: attention and listening / topic vocabulary

## Focus activities

## Character game

The practitioner should go through different kinds of Egyptian people and their roles . . . pictures would be useful to accompany this. Emphasise the 'who' component as you discuss.

The children then walk around the room . . . when the practitioner shouts out a person, they need to act out this person. All decide at the start how each character may present using describing vocabulary.

*The Pharaoh* had the most power. He was responsible for making laws and keeping order, ensuring that Egypt was safe.

(Strong, powerful, stern, scary, daunting, rich etc.)

*The Vizier* was the Pharaoh's chief advisor.

(Clever, powerful etc.)

*Nobles* ruled areas of Egypt. They were responsible for making local laws and keeping order in their area.

(Brave, strong, scary)

*Scribes* were the only people who could read and write and were responsible for keeping records.

(Intelligent, clever, carry around books, pens)

*Soldiers* were responsible for defending the country.

(Brave, strong, courageous, carried weapons, wore armour)

*Craftsmen* were skilled workers, such as pottery makers, leatherworkers, sculptors, painters, weavers, jewellery makers, shoemakers.

(Clever, creative, patient, used their hands, sculpt, paint, weave, use tools)

*Farmers* worked the land of the Pharaoh and Nobles and were given housing, food and clothes in return.

(Hardworking, strong, dirty, dig, sow seeds)

*Slaves* were usually prisoners captured in war. Slaves could be found in the house of the Pharaoh and Nobles, working in mines and in temples.

(Poor, old clothes and rags, hardworking, scrubbed, cleaned, cooked)

Extend: tap a child on the shoulder and get the child to add dialogue to his or her acting . . . what might the character be saying/thinking.

Once the child has said his or her sentence out loud, everyone else copies what the child said verbatim as they are acting.

E.g. Slave: 'I'm so tired and hungry!'. . . Everyone: 'I'm so tired and hungry!'

Developing: attention and listening / processing / describing vocabulary / topic vocabulary / 'who' component / expressive language

## Egyptian shapes

Split children into small groups. The focus of the activity is for children to work together in their group and create shapes of different Egypt-themed items/scenes. They need to communicate together and use their bodies to create the items . . . at the end of the activity, the children can all come together and show the others some of their creations.

It would be useful for pictures to accompany the words given to the children, as some of this vocabulary will be brand new . . .

Items/scenes that can be given to the groups to create:

Pyramid

Sphinx

River Nile

Tomb

Valley of the Kings

Tutankhamen

Hieroglyphics

Archaeologists

(other topic-related vocabulary they may be studying in class)

Developing: attention / expressive language / social skills (eye contact, group cohesion, non-verbal communication, negotiation skills) / topic vocabulary

## Egyptian image of the hour

Choose some characters for the children to act out. It could be characters already described in the Egyptian character game or characters from an Egyptian-themed story they are covering or general Egyptian-themed characters: Cleopatra, Howard Carter, Tutankhamen, etc.

The children walk around the room, and when the practitioner shouts 'freeze,' they all stop. The practitioner then shouts out a character and a time. . . . The children have to act out the character and what they would be doing at that time and then another character or time so there is a contrast. . . .

For example:

The practitioner shouts out 'Freeze . . . Slave at 10 p.m.' (children act out working, clearing up etc.). The practitioner then shouts out, 'Pharaoh at 10 p.m.!' (children act out sleeping or perhaps eating and drinking . . .).

The practitioner shouts out, 'Freeze . . . Howard Carter at 2 p.m.' (children act out searching, dusting off artefacts etc.).

The practitioner then shouts out, 'Howard Carter at 10 p.m.!' (children act out sleeping or perhaps reading . . .).

Developing: attention and listening / processing / comprehension / time vocabulary and concept / 'when' component / 'who' component / topic vocabulary

## Howard Carter tomb escape

One child is blindfolded and stands at one end of the room – that child is 'Howard Carter.'

Tell the children that Howard Carter needs to escape from the tomb . . . other children are placed around the room in various spots – they are the 'Mummies.'

These children can move two steps in any direction from their original spot and back . . . but no further . . .

Another child then has to help Howard Carter find his way to the other side of the room without being grabbed by one of the Mummies.

The child giving the instructions should use directional language (forwards, side step, turn left, right, diagonal etc.).

If a child is touched by one of the Mummies, they are out, and the instructor is out, and the Mummy has a go with the blindfold on.

Take turns with different children being blindfolded and giving instructions.

Developing: attention and listening / following and giving instructions / direction concepts use and understanding / social skills (partner cohesion and trust / listening to peers / taking turns) / topic vocabulary

## Tomb challenge

The practitioner puts some rows of tables together (the number of rows depends on the number of teams there are) and covers them with blankets or sheets if possible to make it dark (if not, children can pretend); this is to represent climbing into a dark tomb . . .

The children are to be split into small groups of around three.

The children are to pretend they are Howard Carter and his team of archaeologists and they are going into Tutankhamen's tomb to discover what is in there.

Firstly the team need to pack a bag of things they will need . . . they are going to be away from their camp for three days . . . what will they need?

The children decide in groups, what to pack? Prepare them by thinking about weather in day and night in the desert. What will they need to eat and drink? How will they sleep? What will they need for their search in the dark tomb?

Once they describe what is in their bags, they go to the entrance of their tomb. . . . The rules are that they can only go in (under the table and out to other side) one at a time per team, and they have to remember *three* artefacts they see. . . . They can't move them as they don't want to damage them.

The practitioner should lay out a variety of pictures of artefacts and their label (see Internet for these and print them off and cut them out) on the other side of the table (tomb).

Each child goes under the table and crawls through to the end. They need to remember three artefacts and then crawl back through to their team and tell them the three things . . .

One of the children writes this down. Then the next archaeologist goes in and again memorises three artefacts (different to the ones others have said) and then comes back and reports what he or she has found.

The teams are timed with a stopwatch and have five minutes to discover and list as many artefacts as they can.

The children should only discover *three* artefacts at a time and tell them that there is a poison gas that is in the tomb so they only have time for three artefacts at a time!

Examples of artefacts that can be used: vases / gold / silver / jewels / jewellery / headdress / chariot / chair / throne / coffin / statues / perfume / oils / food / wine / weapons / shields / musical instruments / ornaments.

The winning team is the team with the most artefacts

Developing: attention and listening / memory / topic vocabulary / social skills (group cohesion / listening to each other / eye contact / assigning roles and working together) / conversation skills / negotiation / verbal reasoning / prediction / expressive language skills

## Story square

Acting out a story with an Ancient Egypt theme:

For example:

- The Egyptian Cinderella (by Shirley Climo)

- Croco'nile' (by Roy Gerrard)

- The Story of Cleopatra[4]

- The Time Travelling Cat and the Egyptian Goddess (by Julia Jarman)

- Flat Stanley – The Great Egyptian Grave Robbery (by Jeff Brown)

Some of the focus activities listed can be changed to suit the: 'who,' 'where' and 'when' elements of the Egyptian-themed story chosen to help embed the story further.

Developing: attention and listening / story understanding / narrative development / processing / comprehension / spoken language recall / expressive language / social skills (eye contact / communication with others / sharing space and cooperation / non-verbal communication)

## Curators

The children are put into small groups and told they are curators (define this word for them) at a museum. Each group is given three pictures of artefacts (these can be easily sourced from the Internet). They have to work in their groups together and come up with a story behind each artefact. . . . It can be completely fictitious.

Story components should be out for them to use and guide their description:

Who used the artefact?

Where was it found?

When was it used? (e.g. 250 BCE)

What was it used for?

Why did it stop being used? (the end)

The groups should be supported where needed by the practitioner. Children should be encouraged to make sure everyone in the group has at least one idea put into the story.

They should also be encouraged to reflect on the ancient Egypt knowledge they have and use this to help their stories.

To differentiate and make it easier for those that need it, provide pictures/labels next to the story components.

(Who: Cleopatra, Tutankhamen, Pharaohs, Soldier, Scribe, Farmer, Slave etc.)

(Where: pyramid / tomb / Valley of the Kings / River Nile / Egypt)

(When: 250 BCE / 50 BCE / 2000 BCE)

And so on . . .

Once the groups have developed their stories, they take on the role of curators, and the three pictures are spread out across the room. They then present the items, names and stories to the museum visitors (other children from other groups) and guide them along the room as they talk.

Each group has a turn at this.

Evaluate at the end – ask other children to comment / remember facts about the other group's artefacts.

Developing: attention / topic vocabulary / social skills (turn taking / group cohesion / negotiation / prediction / conversation skills) / expressive language / verbal reasoning / memory / presentation skills / comprehension

## The story of Cleopatra

There was once a princess of Egypt called Cleopatra. Her father was the Pharaoh, and he was called Ptolemy the 7th (pronounced: Tol-emy). Cleopatra was his favourite child. Cleopatra was a very clever child, and she learned a lot about the country and how her father ruled it. Cleopatra learned many languages including Greek, Egyptian and Latin. When Cleopatra was 18 years old, her father died. He left the throne to both her and her younger brother, who was 10 years old, and he was called Ptolemy the 8th.

Cleopatra and her brother got married because this was a tradition in those times.

They were to rule Egypt as co-rulers together.

Cleopatra was much older than her brother, and she became the main ruler of Egypt. She was a very good ruler.

However, as her brother Ptolemy got older, he wanted more power. Eventually he forced Cleopatra from the palace, and as the main ruler he became the Pharaoh.

One day Julius Caesar, who was a Roman Emperor, came from Rome and arrived in Egypt. Cleopatra snuck back into the palace hidden inside a rolled up carpet. She met with Caesar and convinced him to help her take the throne back for herself.

Caesar's army fought with Ptolemy's army at the 'Battle of Nile.' Caesar's army defeated Ptolemy's army.

Ptolemy drowned and died in the River Nile, and Cleopatra became the Pharaoh of Egypt.

The people of Egypt liked Cleopatra, and she was seen as a very good ruler. The country was successful during her rule.

After the battle between Caesar and Ptolemy, Cleopatra and Julius Caesar fell in love. They had a child named Caesarion. Cleopatra visited Rome and lived there.

Julius Caesar was assassinated in Rome, and Cleopatra returned to Egypt.

A leader called Marc Antony came into power after Caesar was killed, and Cleopatra and Marc Antony met and fell in love.

They brought their armies together and set them against another of Rome's leaders who was called Octavian. Octavian was the son of Julius Caesar and his heir. Cleopatra wanted her son, Caesarion, to be Caesar's heir and to eventually become ruler of Rome.

Cleopatra and Marc Antony combined their armies in order to fight Octavian. The two armies met and fought.

Antony and Cleopatra were defeated by Octavian and had to go back to Egypt.

Marc Antony returned to the battlefield hoping to defeat Octavian. He was not winning and realised that he was going to be defeated and captured by Octavian.

Marc Antony was then told the false news that Cleopatra had died. Antony killed himself.

Cleopatra was devastated, and some say she killed herself by allowing a poisonous snake to bite her.

Cleopatra and Marc Antony were buried side by side as Cleopatra had wished.

With Cleopatra's death, Octavian took control of Egypt, and it became part of the Roman Empire. Her death brought an end the Egyptian Empire, and she was the last Pharaoh of Egypt.

## Notes

1  See Appendix D for punctuation symbols which can be photocopied
2  Excellent website for pictorial resources to use: www.twinkl.co.uk: search 'Romans'
3  Excellent website for pictorial resources to use: www.twinkl.co.uk: search 'Egypt'
4  See Appendix E for this story – a simple version has been written by author from using various sources and can be acted out in the story square

# Appendix A
# EVALUATIONS

## General Session Evaluation: Reception and Key Stage 1

Session Number:  Story Session Title:

Pupils in Session:

| Area of Speech, Language and Communication Targeted | Tick if Targeted |
|---|---|
| **Non-verbal Skills:** | |
| Attention | |
| Listening | |
| Non-verbal communication / facial expression | |
| **Receptive Language Areas / Memory / Processing** | |
| Following instructions (within activity) | |
| Understanding question words . . . List question words targeted: | |
| Understanding descriptions (e.g. following practitioner descriptions in activities) | |
| Memory | |
| Processing | |
| **Expressive Language (Verbal)** | |
| Using complete sentences | |
| Using question words . . . List question words targeted: | |
| Recalling sentences verbatim | |
| Sequencing | |
| **Phonological Awareness** | |
| Areas of phonological awareness worked on: | |

| Higher-Level Language | |
|---|---|
| Verbal reasoning | |
| Answering why / what if / how questions | |
| Prediction | |
| Inference | |

| Narrative Skills | |
|---|---|
| Understanding story in story square | |
| Story components covered in discussion: who, where, when, what, the end | |
| Contributing to story making | |
| Story components directly covered in activities: who, where, when, what, the end | |

| Vocabulary | |
|---|---|
| Description vocabulary / concepts / feelings vocabulary within session: | |
| Topic/story vocabulary targeted in session: | |

| Social Skills / Pragmatics | |
|---|---|
| Turn taking | |
| Eye contact | |
| Conversation skills | |
| Social language (greetings, ending conversations etc.) | |
| Negotiation | |
| Tolerance | |
| Teamwork / cohesion | |

**Areas Targeted Not Listed:**

**Additional Comments / Notes:**

**Date:**                                        **Signed:**

## Single Pupil Evaluation: Reception and Key Stage 1

Session Number:                    Name of Pupil:

Story Session Title:

| Area of Speech, Language and Communication Targeted | Tick if Targeted | Tick if achieved |
|---|---|---|
| Story components covered in activities (who, where, when, what, end) | | |
| **Non-verbal Skills:** | | |
| Attention | | |
| Listening | | |
| Non-verbal communication / facial expression | | |
| **Receptive Language Areas / Memory/ Processing** | | |
| Following instructions (within activity) | | |
| Understanding story components / question words (shown within completion section)<br><br>Who:<br><br>Where:<br><br>When:<br><br>What:<br><br>The end: | | |
| Understanding stories/descriptions | | |
| Memory | | |

| Expressive Language (Verbal) | | |
|---|---|---|
| Using complete sentences | | |
| Question words used (asking questions) | | |
| Recalling sentences verbatim<br>Number of words could recall in a sentence: | | |
| Sequencing | | |
| **Phonological Awareness** | | |
| Rhyme | | |
| Initial sound | | |
| **Higher-Level Language** | | |
| Verbal reasoning | | |
| Answering why / what if / how questions | | |
| Prediction | | |
| Inference | | |
| **Vocabulary** | | |
| Description vocabulary / concepts / feelings vocabulary within session:<br>List any specifically used by child independently: | | |
| Topic/story vocabulary in session:<br>Also list any vocabulary the child specifically used independently: | | |

| Social Skills / Pragmatics | | |
|---|---|---|
| Turn taking | | |
| Eye contact | | |
| Conversation skills | | |
| Social language (greetings, ending conversations etc.) | | |
| Negotiation | | |
| Tolerance/patience | | |
| Teamwork/cohesion | | |

Any other comments / areas to focus on next session:

**Date:**                                    **Signed:**

© 2018, *Developing Children's Speech, Language and Communication through Stories and Drama*, Jodi Lea-Trowman, Routledge

## Session Evaluation: Key Stage 2

**Session Number:**                    **Session Title:**

**Pupils in Session:**

| Activity Chosen | SLCN Targeted:<br>List Area Targeted and Vocabulary /<br>Concepts/ Language Covered |
|---|---|
| **Introduction:** | |
| | |
| **Warm Up:** | |
| | |
| **Focus One:** | |
| | |

## Focus Two:

## Completion:

## Additional Comments:

**Date:**                    **Signed:**

## Single Pupil Evaluation: Key Stage 2

**Session Number:**      **Session Title:**

**Pupil:**

| Activity Delivered | SLCN Targeted |
| --- | --- |
| | **Comments on Student Participation** |

### Introduction:

| | |
| --- | --- |
| | |
| | |

### Warm Up:

| | |
| --- | --- |
| | |
| | |

### Focus One:

| | |
| --- | --- |
| | |
| | |

**Focus Two:**

**Completion:**

**Additional Comments:**

**Date:**                                              **Signed:**

# Appendix B
# EVALUATION EXAMPLES

| Session Evaluation: Reception and Key Stage 1 (example) | |
|---|---|
| Session Number:          5 Story Session Title: Rainbow Fish session one | |
| Pupils in Session: Ellen, Anthony, Tammy, John, Gemma, Gregory, Elizabeth, Paul, Kate, Celine | |
| **Area of Speech, Language and Communication Targeted** | **Tick if Targeted** |
| **Non-verbal Skills:** | |
| Attention | ✓ |
| Listening | ✓ |
| Non-verbal communication / facial expression | ✓ |
| **Receptive Language Areas / Memory / Processing** | |
| Following instructions (within activity) | |
| Understanding question words . . . List question words targeted<br>Who – children asked, who are you? | ✓ |
| Understanding descriptions (e.g. following practitioner descriptions in activities)<br>Followed description for journey to story square | ✓ |
| Memory | |
| Processing | ✓ |
| **Expressive Language (Verbal)** | |
| Using complete sentences | ✓ |
| Using questions words . . . List question words targeted:<br>Hot-seat activity – children using how/what questions | |
| Recalling sentences verbatim | ✓ |
| Sequencing | ✓ |

| Phonological Awareness | |
|---|---|
| Areas of phonological awareness worked on: | |

| Higher-Level Language | |
|---|---|
| Verbal reasoning | ✓ |
| Answering why / what if / how questions<br>Hot-seat: Paul and Elizabeth octopus today . . . answered how questions | ✓ |
| Prediction: Tammy unable to predict story from pictures | ✓ |
| Inference | |

| Narrative Skills | |
|---|---|
| Understanding story in story square | ✓ |
| Story components covered in discussion: who, where, when, what, the end<br>Anthony and Ellen losing focus in this task | ✓ |
| Contributing to story making | |
| Story components directly covered in activities: who, where, when, what, the end<br>Who – ocean creatures | ✓ |

| Vocabulary | |
|---|---|
| Description vocabulary/concepts/feelings vocabulary within session:<br><br>Actions and describing vocabulary around sea creatures<br><br>Feelings vocabulary | |
| Topic/story vocabulary targeted in session:<br><br>Ocean creatures vocabulary<br><br>Advice | |

| Social Skills / Pragmatics | | |
|---|---|---|
| Turn taking:  Gemma needs prompts with this at times | | ✓ |
| Eye contact | | ✓ |
| Conversation skills | | ✓ |
| Social language (greetings, ending conversations etc.) | | ✓ |
| Negotiation | | |
| Tolerance | | |
| Teamwork/cohesion | | ✓ |

**Areas Targeted Not Listed:**
Playground rehearsal . . . can I play with you?
Discussion about sharing

**Additional Comments/Notes:**
Rainbow Fish session two next session
Excellent attention today
Gregory and Ellen answered who, where and when about story today
Children all using 'Can I play?' sentence, and all gave good feedback about this at the end. . . . Kate needs some work around social skills at times
Repeat this game in class later this week.
Octopus hot-seat activity started . . . needs to be completed with more children being octopus in role

Date: 30-09-17  Signed: J Lea-Trowman

| Single Pupil Evaluation: Reception and Key Stage 1 | | |
|---|---|---|
| Session number: 4 and 5 | | Name of pupil: Sunny |
| Story Session Title: Handa's Surprise session 1 and Handa's Surprise session 2 | | |

| Area of Speech, Language and Communication Targeted | Tick if Targeted | Tick if Achieved |
|---|---|---|
| Story components covered in activities (who, where, when, what, end): Who, where | | |
| **Non-verbal Skills:** | | |
| Attention | ✓ | ✓ |
| Listening | ✓ | ✓ |
| Non-verbal communication / facial expression<br>Good pretending to be surprised opening pretend box | ✓ | ✓ |

| Receptive Language Areas / Memory / Processing | | |
|---|---|---|
| Following instructions (within activity) | | |
| Understanding story components / question words (shown within completion section)<br>Who: answered Monkey for who | ✓ | ✓ |
| Where: answered 'Africa' during completion. Good as progress as she couldn't originally predict Africa when story first introduced. | ✓ | ✓ |
| When: unable to answer when | ✓ | ✓ |
| What: not seen | ✓ | |
| The end: | ✓ | |
| Understanding stories/descriptions<br>Guessed a child gift through its description correctly | ✓ | ✓ |
| Good participation in story square activity and used some question-mark actions in correct places | | |
| Memory<br>Could not remember what gift the child next to her had received | ✓ | |
| **Expressive Language (Verbal)** | | |
| Using complete sentences<br>Sunny described pretend gift: 'It's something to eat and it's round and it's a fruit . . . it's green.' | ✓ | ✓ |
| Question words *used* (asking questions) | | |
| Recalling sentences verbatim<br>Number of words could recall in a sentence:<br>Repeated back sentence<br>'Will she like this soft yellow banana' – 7 words | ✓ | ✓ |
| Sequencing | | |
| **Phonological Awareness** | | |
| Rhyme | | |
| Initial sound | | |
| **Higher-Level Language** | | |
| Verbal reasoning | | |
| Answering why / what if / how questions<br>Unable to answer why question | ✓ | |
| Prediction<br>Couldn't answer what they think story was about or where it was | ✓ | |
| Inference | | |

| Vocabulary | | |
|---|---|---|
| Description vocabulary /concepts / feelings vocabulary within session:<br>List any specifically used by child independently:<br>Tall                          Heavy/light<br>Long<br>Thin                          synonyms for hot and cold<br>Fast<br>Big              stomping              peek<br>cheeky<br>peck         slow         stripey         open<br>Sunny generated thin and stomping independently<br>Generated synonym: boiling | ✓ | ✓ |
| Topic/story vocabulary in session:<br>Also list any vocabulary the child specifically used independently:<br>All fruit vocab found in story with corresponding animal<br><br>Clothes vocabulary – named t-shirt for hot weather and hat for cold weather<br>Sunny said zebra, monkey and mango independently<br>Could differentiate between healthy and non-healthy foods | ✓ | ✓ |

| Social Skills / Pragmatics | | |
|---|---|---|
| Turn taking | ✓ | ✓ |
| Eye contact | | |
| Conversation skills | | |
| Social language (greetings, ending conversations etc.) | | |
| Negotiation | | |
| Tolerance/patience | | |
| Teamwork/cohesion | | |

Any other comments / areas to focus on next session:
Doesn't understand 'when' . . . confidence improving . . . work on social skills more next sessions. Next book the class are reading: Gingerbread Man.

Date: 10-09-2017                                        Signed: J Lea-Trowman

## Session Evaluation: Key Stage 2

**Session Number**: 4        **Session Title**: Romans Session 4

**Pupils in Session**: Carly, Amanda, Abbie, Zoe, Anna, Claire

| Activity Delivered | SLCN Targeted |
|---|---|
| | Comments on Student Participation |
| **Introduction:** | |
| Recap on who: the different types of roman roles: emperor, slave etc. . . . <br><br> Where: different places Romans used: baths, markets, homes, amphitheatres <br><br> When: recap on meaning of BCE and CE <br><br> What happened in story Romulus and Remus | Narrative elements to help recap: who, where, when, what happened? <br> Review and recap language from previous sessions <br> Sentences around the topic |
| | All named a Roman role or famous character <br> Abbie and Anna struggled with recall of BCE and CE <br> All retold elements of Romulus and Remus together |
| **Warm Up:** | |
| Months of the year line up <br><br> Carried out twice: (as 6 students) <br> Jan to June first time <br> July to Dec second time | Attention <br> Social skills: turn taking, collaboration, tolerance, patience, eye contact, non-verbal comm, group cohesion <br> Months of the year vocabulary and sequencing <br> 'when' component |
| | Zoe and Anna needed peer support with where to stand in months activity |
| **Focus One:** | |
| Roman towns | Attention and listening <br> Processing <br> 'Where' component <br> British places vocabulary <br><br> All enjoyed game – at the end each student could name one place that had a Roman 'ending' on its name. |

| **Focus Two:** | |
|---|---|
| Hadrian's Fact Hunt | Attention and listening<br>Processing<br>Memory<br>Comprehension<br>Vocabulary<br>Social skills: turn taking, eye contact, starting and finishing an interaction<br>'What' component |
| | Abbie had fact written down to aid memory. Others remembered facts.<br><br>Enjoyed mixing and social skills good<br><br>All could name one other fact at the end of activity – however, Zoe needed some prompting from peer to remember length of wall . . . |

| **Completion:** | |
|---|---|
| Recap and shake off session | De-roll |
| | All named a British place<br>Recited months of the year all together (to help support those who are still unsure)<br>All said their own Hadrian's Wall fact |

| **Additional Comments:** |
|---|
| Do a BCE/CE activity next week to embed this further . . . another months-of-the-year activity if possible – do timeline activity Introduce Roman numerals as covering this in class this next week Do another Hadrian's Wall activity to embed Anna, Zoe and Abbie need more support |

Date: 20-02-17                                    Signed: J Lea-Trowman

| Single Pupil Evaluation: Key Stage 2 | |
|---|---|
| **Session Number**:     8 | **Session Title**: Worst Witch (by Jill Murphy) session 2 |
| **Pupil**: Sarah | |
| **Activity Delivered** | **SLCN Targeted** |
| | **Comments on Student Participation** |
| **Introduction:** | |
| Recap on Worst Witch<br>Who are main characters<br>Where it is set<br>When<br>What happens in first chapter<br><br>Introduce current session and look at chapter 2 | Recap/review<br><br>Intro to chapter 2 |
| | Could remember some characters:<br>Mildred, Ethel and Ms Cackle and named the Academy<br>Could not join in with the main aspects of what happened in chapter 1 |
| **Warm Up:** | |
| Alliteration names<br><br>Students to think of an adjective first time round, then a verb second time round . . .<br><br>Extended so that they had to think of a character from book and do alliteration . . . | Attention and listening<br>Phonological awareness: initial sound<br>Alliteration knowledge and use<br>Processing and imitation |
| | Excellent – joined in and repeated others contributions – came up with own adjective and verb:<br>Slimey Sarah<br>Starjump Sarah<br><br>Couldn't think of another character as other students had already taken the ones she knew . . . Practitioner reminded her of character 'Drusilla'<br>She then did: 'Deadly Drusilla!' . . . excellent! |

| **Focus One:** | |
|---|---|
| Guess the noun<br>From passage in chapter 2<br>E.g. 'The presentation took place in the great . . .'<br><br>Repeated the four pages done in 'guess the noun' and acted out in story square | Attention and listening<br>Comprehension<br>Processing<br>Noun awareness<br>Inference<br>Prediction<br>Familiarity with chapter 2<br>Story square skills<br>Guessed some correctly<br>Needed repetition of sentences 2 or 3 times.<br><br>Story square: Sarah imitated a line correctly and understood story as she acted out different roles: table, Miss Cackle, kitten |
| **Focus Two:** | |
| Hot seat<br>Character: Miss Hardbroom: Deputy Head – played by practitioner<br><br>Asking about her own school<br>What kind of student was she<br>Finding out why she is so strict and mean sometimes . . .<br>Life experiences<br>What are her punishments?<br>Does she like any of the students?<br>Who doesn't she like?<br>Why?<br>Etc. . . . | Attention / asking questions / expressive language |
| | Asked who Miss Hardbroom does not like and remembered to follow this up with the question 'why' |
| **Completion:** | |
| Review session<br><br>De-roll | Review and recap story<br>Use of story components<br>Recap elements of chapter 2 in particular<br>De-roll |
| | All students could recall 'who' appeared in chapter 2 and 'where' the scene was" |

**Additional Comments:**

Excellent participation – needs some repetition at times.
Recap and reviews very important for Sarah
Next week focusing on parts of what Miss Hardbroom said in her answers to create
a short story on Miss Hardbroom when she was at school . . . Sarah will need lots of
recap on what hot-seat answers were today

Date: 07-10-17                    Signed: J-Lea-Trowman

# Appendix C

# PRE- AND POST-ASSESSMENT FORMS

| Name of student:<br>Date checklist completed 1:<br>Date checklist completed 2: | | | |
|---|---|---|---|
| | **1** | **2** | **3** |
| **Area of Speech, Language and Communication** | **Not Achieved** | **Partially Achieved** | **Achieved** |
| Attention (child able to attend for majority of activity) | | | |
| Listening (child showing listening skills in tasks) | | | |
| Non-verbal communication / facial expression (appropriate use of NV communication and facial expressions within activities requiring this) | | | |
| Following instructions (within an activity – not in general) | | | |
| Understanding story components / question words:<br><br>Who:<br><br>Where:<br><br>When:<br><br>What:<br><br>The end: | | | |
| Understanding stories/descriptions (follows a story and can act out what they hear) | | | |
| Memory (can child remember simple words / sentences / responses of others) | | | |
| Child uses complete sentences | | | |

| | | | |
|---|---|---|---|
| Use of question words: is child able to ask questions starting with:<br><br>Who<br><br>Where<br><br>When<br><br>What<br><br>How | | | |
| Can child recall most sentences verbatim | | | |
| Sequencing (can child sequence events in order) | | | |
| Rhyme (can child generate rhyming words) | | | |
| Initial sound (can child generate a word with a given initial sound) | | | |
| Can child answer higher-level questions:<br><br>Why:<br><br>What if:<br><br>How questions: | | | |
| Prediction (can child make a prediction using language) | | | |
| Inference (can child make inferences from language: e.g. not be directly told but to infer from a description what is happening) | | | |
| Use of description vocabulary / concepts / feelings vocabulary:<br>(does child use these consistently within descriptions) | | | |
| Turn taking (can child take turns appropriately) | | | |
| Eye contact (can child make eye contact appropriately) | | | |
| Conversation skills (can child engage in conversation with a peer) | | | |
| Social language (can child use greetings / enter conversations / end conversations appropriately) | | | |
| Negotiation (can child use persuasive language with peers) | | | |

| | | | |
|---|---|---|---|
| Tolerance/patience (can child wait for others appropriately) | | | |
| Team cohesion (can child work within a group appropriately) | | | |
| **Scores** | | | |
| Total Assessment One: | | | |
| Total Assessment Two: | | | |

**Total Overall Assessment One =**

**Total Overall Assessment Two =**

| Name of Student: Nikki | Date Checklist Completed 1: 25-09-16<br>Date Checklist Completed 2: 15-05-17 | | |
|---|---|---|---|
| | 1 | 2 | 3 |
| **Area of Speech, Language and Communication** | **Not Achieved** | **Partially Achieved** | **Achieved** |
| Attention (child able to attend for majority of activity) | | ✓ | ✓ |
| Listening (child showing listening skills in tasks) | | ✓✓ | |
| Non-verbal communication / facial expression (appropriate use of NV communication and facial expressions within activities requiring this) | | | ✓✓ |
| Following instructions (within an activity – not in general) | | ✓✓ | |
| Understanding story components / question words: | | | |
| Who: | ✓ | ✓ | ✓✓ |
| Where: | ✓ | ✓ | ✓ |
| When: | | ✓ | ✓ |
| What: | | | ✓ |
| The end: | | | |
| Understanding stories/descriptions (follows a story and can act out what they hear) | | ✓ | ✓ |
| Memory (can child remember simple words / sentences / responses of others) | | ✓✓ | |
| Child uses complete sentences | | ✓ | ✓ |
| Use of question words: is child able to ask questions starting with: | | | |
| Who | ✓ | ✓ | ✓✓ |
| Where | ✓ | ✓ | ✓ |
| When | | ✓ | ✓ |
| What | | | ✓ |
| How | | | |

| | | | |
|---|---|---|---|
| Can child recall most sentences verbatim | | ✓ | ✓ |
| Sequencing (can child sequence events in order) | | ✓ | ✓ |
| Rhyme (can child generate rhyming words) | | ✓ | ✓ |
| Initial sound (can child generate a word with a given initial sound) | ✓ | ✓ | |
| Can child answer higher-level questions:<br><br>Why:<br><br>What if:<br><br>How questions: | ✓<br><br>✓✓<br><br>✓ | ✓<br><br>✓ | |
| Prediction (can child make a prediction using language) | | ✓ | ✓ |
| Inference (can child make inferences from language: e.g. not be directly told but to infer from a description what is happening) | | ✓✓ | |
| Use of description vocabulary / concepts / feelings vocabulary:<br>(does child use these consistently within descriptions) | | ✓ | ✓ |
| Turn taking (can child take turns appropriately) | | ✓ | ✓ |
| Eye contact (can child make eye contact appropriately) | | ✓✓ | |
| Conversation skills (can child engage in conversation with a peer) | ✓ | ✓ | |
| Social language (can child use greetings / enter conversations / end conversations appropriately) | ✓ | ✓ | |
| Negotiation (can child use persuasive language with peers) | ✓ | ✓ | |
| Tolerance/patience (can child wait for others appropriately) | | ✓ | ✓ |
| Team cohesion (can child work within a group appropriately) | | ✓ | ✓ |
| **Scores** | | | |
| **Total Assessment One:** | 11 | 38 | 12 |
| **Total Assessment Two:** | 1 | 28 | 57 |

**Total Overall Assessment One = 61**

**Total Overall Assessment Two = 86**

# Appendix D
# PUNCTUATION SYMBOLS

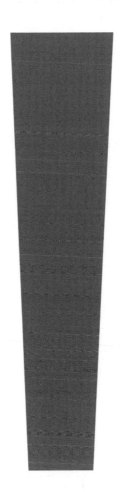

EXCLAMATION MARK

SPEECH MARKS

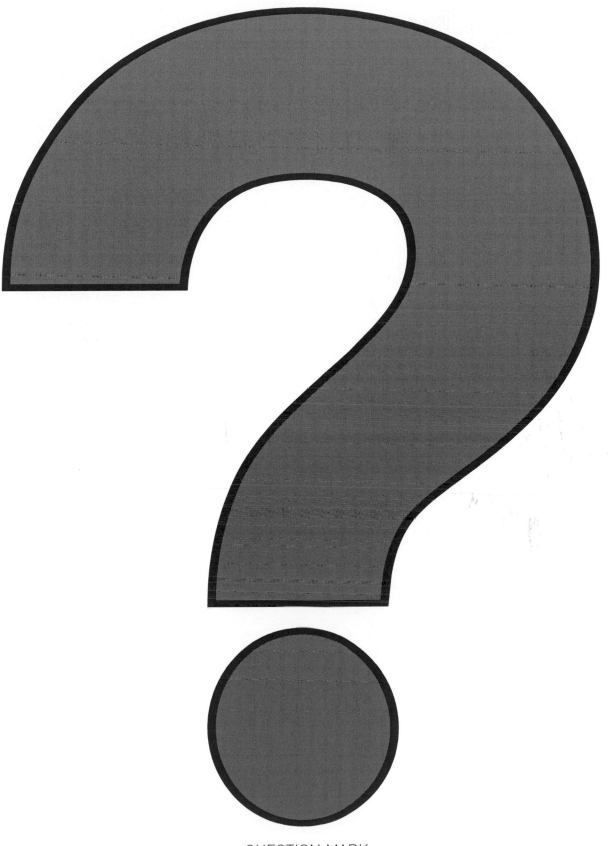

QUESTION MARK

# Appendix E
# STORY COMPONENT CARDS

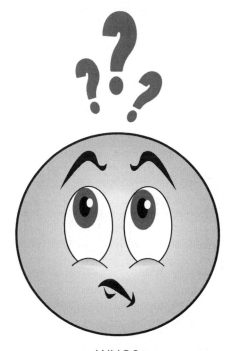

WHO?

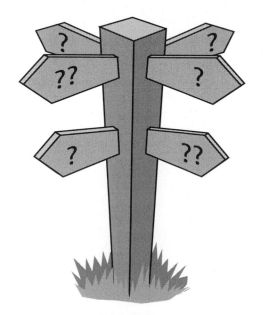

WHERE?

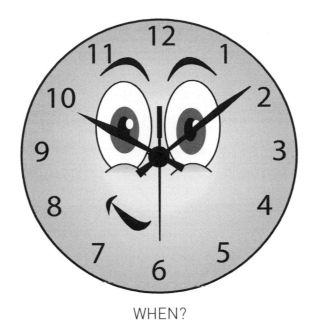

WHEN?

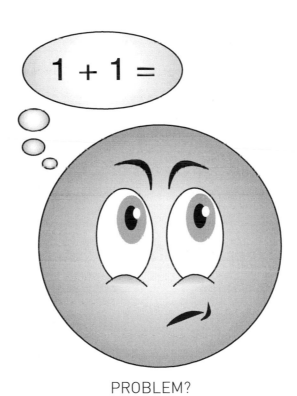

PROBLEM?

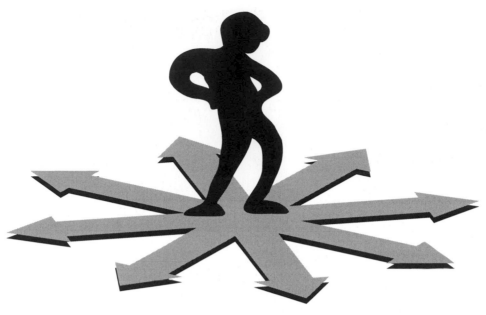

WHAT?

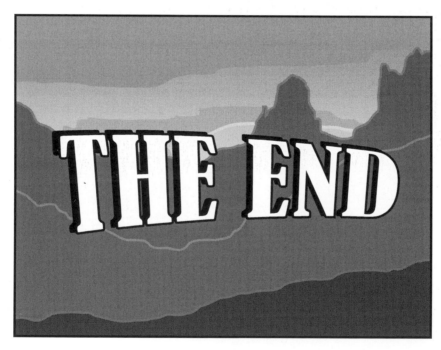

THE END

**WHEN**

**WHO**

**WHERE**

**PROBLEM**

**WHAT**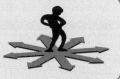

**THE END**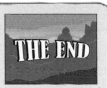

*DESCRIBE*

# BIBLIOGRAPHY

Adams, C., Coke, R., Crutchley, A., Hesketh, A., and Reeves, D. (2001). *Assessment of Comprehension and Expression 6–11 Years*. GL Assessment.

Allan, L. and Leitão, S. (2004). *Peter and the Cat Narrative Assessment*. Black Sheep Press.

Bangles. (1986). *Walk Like an Egyptian*. Columbia Records.

Blank, M., Rose, S.A., and Berlin, L.J. (1978). *The Language of Learning: The Pre-School Years*. Grune & Stratton.

Boal, A. (1979). *Theatre of the Oppressed*. Pluto Press.

Boal, A. (1994). *The Rainbow of Desire: The Boal Method of Theatre and Therapy*. Routledge.

Bolten, G. and Heathcote, D. (1995). *Drama for Learning: Dorothy Heathcote's Mantle of the Expert Approach to Education*. Pearson Education.

Bowell, P. and Heap, B. (2001). *Planning Process Drama*. David Fulton.

Bruner, J.S. (1996). *The Culture of Education*. Harvard University Press.

Carey, J. (2006). *Squirrel Story Narrative Assessment*. Black Sheep Press.

Clipson-Boyles, S. (2012). *Teaching Primary English Through Drama: A Practical and Creative Approach*. Routledge.

Communication Trust: Progression Tool. Available at: www.thecommunicationtrust.org.uk/resources/resources/resources-for-practitioners/progression-tools-primary/

Corbett, P. and Strong, J. (2011). *Talk for Writing Across the Curriculum*. Open University Press.

Department for Education. (2013). The national curriculum in England. Key stages 1 and 2 framework document. Crown Copyright.

Department for Education. (2014). Statutory framework for the early years foundation stage. Setting the standards for learning, development and care for children from birth to five. Crown Copyright. Ref: DFE-00337-2014.

Department for Education and Department for Health. (2015). Special educational needs and disability code of practice: 0 to 25 years. Statutory guidance for organisations, which work with and support children and young people who have special educational needs or disabilities. Crown Copyright.

Farmer, D. (2007). *101 Drama Games and Activities*. Lulu.

Farmer, D. (2012). *Learning Through Drama in the Primary Years*. David Farmer.

Furman, L. (2000). In support of drama in early childhood education, again. *Early Childhood Education Journal*, 27(3), 173–178.

Gersch, I., Haythorne, D., Dix, A., and Leigh, L. (2012). *Dramatherapy With Children, Young People and Schools*. Routledge.

Gussin Paley, V. (1990). *The Boy Who Would Be a Helicopter*. Harvard University Press.

Hughes, M. et al. (2010). Speak Out: Practice Sharing Report. Available at: www.londonbubble.org.uk/uploads/SO_Practice_Sharing_4214.pdf

Kolb, D.A. (1984). *Experiential Learning*. Prentice Hall.

Lee, T. (2011). The Wisdom of Vivian Gussin Paley, in Miller, L. and Pound, L. (eds), *Theories and Approaches to Learning in the Early Years*. Sage Publications.

Mantle of the Expert.com. (2014). Mantle of the Expert.com. Available at: www.mantleoftheexpert.com. [Accessed 25 January 2017].

McMaster, J.C. (1998). 'Doing' literature: Using drama to build literacy. *The Reading Teacher*, 51(7), 574–584.

O'Neill, F. (2007–2009). Evaluation of Speak Out. Available at: www.londonbubble.org.uk/uploads/SO_Evaluation_5371.pdf

PHSE Association. (2016). PHSE Association. Available at: www.pshe-association.org.uk. [Accessed 25 January 2017].

Price, H. (2016). *'Speech Bubbles' Drama Intervention Programme Preliminary Executive Summary of Effectiveness*. Psychological Studies Research Group, School of Social Sciences, UEL.

Taylor, T. (2016). *A Beginners Guide to Mantle of the Expert: A Transformative Approach to Education*. Singular Publishing.

Twinkl Educational Publishing. Available at: www.twinkl.co.uk (Accessed 25th January 2017).

Weldon Johnson, J. (1928). *Dem Bones*. Recorded by Bascomb Lunsford.

Winston, J. (2008). *Beginning Drama 4–11*. David Fulton.

# STORY REFERENCES

Aesop. (1994). *Aesop's Fables*. Wordsworth Children's Classics; New edition (based on original Aesop's Fables).

Ahlberg, J. and Ahlberg, A. (1999). *Funnybones*. Puffin.

Alperin, M. and Latimar, M. (2015). *The Gingerbread Man* (My First Tales). Little Tiger Press (based on folktale: The Ginger Bread Man: Author unknown).

Anderson, H.C. (Bradbury, L. adapter). (1979). *The Ugly Duckling* (Ladybird Well Loved Tales). Ladybird Books Ltd; Reprint edition.

Ashley, B. (2002). *Cleversticks*. Harper Collins Children's Books.

Balit, C. (2005). *Escape From Pompeii*. Frances Lincoln Children's Books; New edition.

Brown, J. (2011). *Flat Stanley: The Great Egyptian Grave Robbery*. Egmont.

Browne, E. (2006). *Handa's Surprise*. Scholastic/Walker Books.

Burningham, J. (1992). *The Shopping Basket*. Red Fox.

Burningham, J. (1994). *Avocado Baby*. Red Fox.

Carle, E. (1994). *The Very Hungry Caterpillar*. Puffin.

Climo, S. (1992). *The Egyptian Cinderella*. Collins; 1st Harper Trophy edition.

Dahl, R. (2016). *George's Marvellous Medicine*. Puffin; New edition.

Davidson, S. (2012). *The Frog Prince*. Usborne Publishing Ltd (based on Brothers Grimm tales: The Frog Prince).

Dodd, L. (2002). *Hairy Maclary From Doladson's Dairy*. Puffin.

Donaldson, J. (2002). *Room on the Broom*. Macmillan Children's Books.

Donaldson, J. (2006). *Rosie's Hat*. Macmillan Children's Books.

Galdone, P. (1981). *The Three Billy Goats Gruff* (Paul Galdone Classics). Houghton Mifflin Co. International Inc.

Gerrard, R. (2001). *Croco'nile*. Farrar Straus Giroux; Reprint edition.

Hughes, S. (2009). *Dogger*. Red Fox; Reprint edition.

Jarman, J. (2006). *The Time Travelling Cant and the Egyptian*. Andersen Press; New edition.

Lear, E. (2012). *The Owl and the Pussycat*. Usborne Publishing Ltd.

Matthews, A. (2010). *Julius Caesar: Shakespeare Stories for Children*. Orchard Books.

Mccaughrean, G. (2001). *Roman Myths: Romulus and Remus*. Orchard Books; New edition.

Murphy, J. (2007). *Whatever Next*. Macmillan Children's Books.

Murphy, J. (2013). *The Worst Witch*. Puffin.

Ottolenghi, C. (2002). *Jack and the Beanstalk*. Brighter Child (based on Jack and the Beanstalk by Benjamin Tabat).

Pfister, M. (2007). *The Rainbow Fish*. North South Books.

Sendak, M. (2000). *Where the Wild Things Are*. Red Fox; New edition.

Tomlinson, J. (2008). *The Owl Who Was Afraid of the Dark*. Egmont; New edition.

Velthuijs, M. (1995). *The Frog and the Stranger*. Anderson Press Ltd.

Waddell, M. (1994). *Owl Babies*. Walker Books Ltd.

Winterfeld, H. (2002). *Detectives in Togas*. Hmh Books fir Young Readers.